Further MCQs For Part 1 FRCR
Multiple Choice Questions with referenced Answers for the Part 1 FRCR Examination

Clare Brenner BA MB BCh BAO
Registrar in Radiology, The Adelaide and Meath Hospital, Dublin.

Samuel Hamilton MA MD FRCR DipMedEd.
Consultant Radiologist, The Adelaide and Meath Hospital, Dublin.

Clinical Press

Copyright: Clinical Press Ltd 1998

All rights reserved. No part of this publication may be reproduced, stored in a retrieval system or transmitted in any form or by any means electronic, mechanical, photocopying or otherwise without the prior permission of the copyright owner.

Whilst the advice and information in this book is believed to be true and accurate at the time of its going to press, neither the authors, the editors, nor the publisher can accept any legal responsibility for any errors or omissions that may be made. The publisher makes no warranty, express or implied, with respect to the material contained herein.

Published by:

Clinical Press Ltd.,
Redland Green Farm,
Redland,
Bristol,
BS6 7HF

Brenner C., Hamilton S.

Further MCQs for Part 1 FRCR

Multiple Choice Questions with referenced Answers for the Part 1 FRCR Examination

Brenner and Hamilton

ISBN 1-85457-038 2

Preface

This is a book of multiple choice questions (MCQs) designed for candidates preparing for the first part of the examination for the Fellowship of the Royal College of Radiologists (FRCR Part 1).

There are five papers, each consisting of sixty questions, each of which has five stems. Each paper is followed by its answers, with relevant references. There may be any combination of true or false answers in each question. Negative marking applies, i.e. minus one for each incorrect answer. The pass mark is 60%, and the time allowed is two hours.

Commonly available textbooks and journals have been used to prepare these questions. We have checked the answers as carefully as possible, but as with all MCQs, there will almost inevitably be debate about some questions, as there often is with the examination itself.

The wording of all questions should be read carefully. There are no hidden meanings and questions should be taken at face value.

This book is not intended as a textbook, but rather as a preparation for forthcoming examinations. Hopefully it will remind candidates of some subjects that they may not have revised, and leave them better prepared.

Samuel Hamilton
Clare Brenner

1998.

ABBREVIATIONS

2D	two dimensional
3D	three dimensional
AP	anteroposterior
C	cervical (spine)
cm(s)	centimetre(s)
CT	computed tomography
DTPA	diethylene triamine pentaacetic acid
HMPAO	hexamethyl propylene amine oxime
keV	kilo electron volt
kV(s)	kilovolt(s)
kVp	peak kilovolt
L	lumbar (spine)
mA	milliampere
mAs	milliampere second
meV	megaelectron volt
mg(s)	milligram(s)
MHz	megahertz
min	minute
ml(s)	millilitre(s)
mm(s)	millimetre(s)
MRI	magnetic resonance imaging
MUGA	multiple gated acquisition
PA	posteroanterior
SPECT	single photon emission computed tomography
STIR	short tau inversion recovery
T	thoracic (spine)
TE	time to echo
TR	time to repeat
Z	atomic number

TEXTBOOKS and JOURNALS

A Textbook of Radiology and Imaging, Sutton, 5th Ed., Churchill Livingstone, 1993.

A Textbook of Radiology and Imaging, Sutton, 6th Ed., Churchill Livingstone, 1997.

A Guide to Radiological Procedures, Chapman & Nakielny, 3rd Ed., Saunders, 1993.

Christensen's Physics of Diagnostic Radiology, Curry et al, 4th Ed., Lea & Febiger, 1990.

Community Radiation Protection Legislation, Commission of the European Communities, 1992.

Gray's Anatomy, 38th Ed., Churchill Livingstone, 1995.

Clark's Positioning in Radiography, Swallow et al, 11th Ed., Heinemann, 1986.

British Journal of Radiology.

Radiographics.

MRI made easy, Schild, Schering, 1990.

Practical Nuclear Medicine, Sharp et al, IRL Press, 1989.

Guidance Notes For The Protection of Persons Against Ionising Radiation Arising From Medical and Dental Use, National Radiation Protection Board, 1988.

Making the best use of a Department of Clinical Radiology; Royal College of Radiologists London, 2nd Ed., 1993.

TEXTBOOKS and JOURNALS (contd.)

An Atlas of Radiological Anatomy, Weir & Abrahams, 2nd Ed., Churchill Livingstone, 1986.

Techniques in Diagnostic Imaging, Whitehouse et al, 2nd Ed., Blackwell Science, 1990.

Ultrasonography in Obstetrics and Gynecology, Callen, 3rd Ed., Saunders, 1994.

Dynamic Radiology of the Abdomen, Meyers, 4th Ed., Springer-Verlag, 1994.

Paper One

Questions

Paper One   Questions

1   In the head and neck

   a)   the carotid sinus is supplied by the glossopharyngeal nerve.
   b)   the carotid sheath contains the internal jugular vein and vagus nerve.
   c)   the external carotid artery has no branches in the neck.
   d)   the lingual artery arises from the internal carotid artery.
   e)   the omohyoid muscle divides the posterior triangle.

2   In embryology of the genito-urinary tract

   a)   the glomeruli develop in the mesonephron.
   b)   the wolffian ducts give rise to the head of the epididymis.
   c)   the collecting ducts develop from the metanephron.
   d)   anomalies of the renal tract occur in 3% of live births.
   e)   horseshoe kidneys fail to migrate upwards due to the superior mesenteric artery.

3   The following are true of the breast

   a)   its base attaches from the second to sixth ribs.
   b)   the superolateral quadrant extends along pectoralis major to the axilla.
   c)   the suspensory stromal ligaments extend from the ducts to the dermis.
   d)   there are 15 to 20 lactiferous ducts.
   e)   the blood supply is via the axillary and internal thoracic arteries only.

4   With regard to endoscopic retrograde cholangiopancreatography (ERCP)

   a)   pancreatic pseudocysts are a contraindication.
   b)   the same density contrast medium is used for biliary and pancreatic duct visualisation.
   c)   acute pancreatitis complicates less than 10% of procedures.
   d)   the biliary tree should be injected first if both biliary and pancreatic ducts are to be demonstrated.
   e)   the right lobe of the liver is commonly underfilled.

5   Lumbar discography

   a)   is indicated in suspected infective discitis.
   b)   is indicated in suspected spondylolisthesis.
   c)   is best performed with contrast medium containing sodium salts.
   d)   requires approximately 1ml of contrast medium for a normal disc.
   e)   requires a higher volume of contrast medium prior to chymopapain therapy.

Paper One Questions

6 In venography

a) high osmolar contrast medium is preferred.
b) a saline flush is not required.
c) non-visualisation of the anterior tibial vein implies pathology.
d) upper limb studies should avoid use of the cephalic vein.
e) the Valsalva manoeuvre may aid diagnosis.

7 Regarding attenuation of an x-ray beam

a) the half value layer is the thickness of absorber needed to halve the original number of photons.
b) the linear attenuation coefficient unit of measurement is the centimetre.
c) the mass attenuation coefficient is independent of the density of the absorber.
d) the linear attenuation coefficient reflects the product of all forms of attenuation.
e) the linear attenuation coefficient applies to polychromatic radiation.

8 Regarding the cranial nerves

a) the optic nerve is the only structure passing through the optic canal.
b) the oculomotor nerve runs in the lateral wall of the cavernous sinus.
c) the maxillary nerve enters the orbit through the inferior orbital fissure.
d) the facial nerve turns forwards at the genicular ganglion.
e) the left recurrent laryngeal nerve arises from the vagus at the level of the subclavian artery.

9 Regarding the laryngeal cartilages

a) the thyroid cartilage has a synovial articulation with the cricoid cartilage.
b) the cricoid cartilage forms a complete ring which is thicker anteriorly.
c) the epiglottis is the only non-hyaline cartilage.
d) the arytenoids give attachment to the true vocal cords.
e) the cartilago triticea lie in the thyrohyoid membrane.

10 Technetium99m

a) is used as the pertechnetate salt.
b) has a half life of six hours.
c) is almost totally excreted by the kidneys.
d) is plasma protein bound.
e) is taken up and secreted by gastric parietal cells.

Paper One   Questions

11 **The following are true of the bladder**

a) its neck is the lowest portion.
b) in men, it is related posteriorly to the seminal vesicles above and the vasa below.
c) in women, the pouch of Douglas separates the bladder and uterus.
d) the medial umbilical ligament arises from its apex.
e) its blood supply arises from the anterior division of the internal iliac.

12 **In the posterior cranial fossa**

a) the medulla oblongata lies in the floor of the fourth ventricle.
b) the basilar artery is closely applied to the pons.
c) the facial nerve nucleus lies in the medulla oblongata.
d) the third ventricle separates the cerebellum from the pons and medulla oblongata.
e) the cerebellar vermis lies below the straight sinus.

13 **Within the atom**

a) a neutral atom has equal numbers of protons and electrons.
b) a K-shell electron has the lowest energy state.
c) a free electron requires energy to remove it from the atom.
d) characteristic x-rays occur when an outer electron moves in towards the nucleus.
e) unfilled shells cause elements to be more stable chemically.

14 **Regarding the vas and spermatic cord**

a) the vas originates at the head of the epididymis.
b) the vas crosses anterior to the external iliac artery and the ureter.
c) an artery to the vas arises from the superior vesical artery.
d) the ejaculatory duct is formed by the union of the vas and the duct of the seminal vesicle.
e) the spermatic cord has three layers of fascia.

15 **For radiographic film**

a) exposure latitude is the exposure range which has useful contrast sensitivity.
b) widening latitude reduces contrast sensitivity.
c) an antihalation layer is used in single emulsion film.
d) the silver halide crystal has a simple cubic structure.
e) reducing latitude reduces contrast sensitivity.

16 Regarding the spleen

a) it is separated from the stomach by the lesser sac.
b) the pleural costodiaphragmatic recess extends to its superior border.
c) the tail of the pancreas, within the lienorenal ligament, lies at the hilum.
d) accessory spleens may occur in the greater omentum and gastrosplenic ligament.
e) the splenic artery divides before entering the hilum.

17 In isotope brain scanning

a) Tc99m pertechnetate has a higher lesion to background uptake than glucoheptonate.
b) Tc99m pertechnetate accumulates in the salivary glands.
c) Tc99m pertechnetate does not cross a damaged blood brain barrier.
d) Tc99m DTPA is used.
e) delayed films are not helpful.

18 In the arterial system

a) the right coronary artery is dominant in 30% of the population.
b) the ulnar artery is usually larger than the radial artery.
c) the gastroduodenal artery arises from the hepatic artery.
d) the superior mesenteric artery lies in front of the splenic vein.
e) the inferior mesenteric artery supplies blood to the lower limbs.

19 A submentovertical view of the skull will show

a) the foramen spinosum.
b) the foramen rotundum.
c) the foramen ovale.
d) the coronoid process of the mandible.
e) the zygomatic arches.

20 In paediatric joint investigation

a) the main indication for hip arthrography in infants is hip dysplasia.
b) septic arthritis is the only major complication of hip arthrography.
c) hip arthrography is performed under local anaesthesia and sedation.
d) hip ultrasound is reliably performed up to six months of age.
e) ultrasound of the hip is performed with a linear array probe of 5 to 7MHz.

Paper One Questions

21 In the venous system

   a) the major draining veins of the heart enter the coronary sinus.
   b) the superior ophthalmic vein connects the facial vein and cavernous sinus.
   c) the external jugular vein lies deep to sternocleidomastoid.
   d) the common carotid artery lies medial to the internal jugular vein.
   e) the inferior petrosal sinus drains into the external jugular vein.

22 In SPECT imaging

   a) standard radionuclides are used.
   b) due to its tomographic nature γ-ray scatter does not degrade the image.
   c) sodium bromide is a typical crystal material.
   d) spatial resolution is largely determined by the collimator.
   e) converging hole collimators have a large field of view.

23 In the upper limb

   a) an os acromiale occurs at the acromial tip in 10% of scapulae.
   b) the conoid tubercle lies on the inferomedial aspect of the clavicle.
   c) the surgical neck of the humerus lies higher than the anatomical neck.
   d) the greater tuberosity is the most lateral part of the proximal humerus.
   e) the coronoid fossa of the humerus lies on its posterior aspect.

24 The following forearm muscles have two heads of origin

   a) pronator teres.
   b) palmaris longus.
   c) flexor carpi ulnaris.
   d) flexor digitorum superficialis.
   e) flexor pollicis longus.

25 In chest radiography

   a) a typical focus-film distance is 300cms for a standard PA view.
   b) a high kV technique improves contrast.
   c) an AP apical view is taken with 30° caudal angulation of the beam.
   d) a lordotic view improves visualisation of the middle lobe.
   e) a single PA film has an effective dose of 0·02 milliSievert.

26 In the small bowel

a) circular folds are more numerous in the ileum than jejunum.
b) lymphatic follicles are larger and more numerous in jejunum than ileum.
c) jejunum and ileum are contained within layers of mesentery.
d) a Meckel's diverticulum may contain pancreatic tissue.
e) circular folds are obliterated with distension of the lumen.

27 In radiographic image quality

a) gray scale appearance depends on the anatomical area being radiographed.
b) gray scale appearance is independent of the radiation exposure.
c) underexposure usually causes an improvement.
d) high contrast film is detrimental to quality in chest radiography.
e) unsharpness causes loss of contrast in an object.

28 In x-ray tubes

a) tube current is independent of filament current.
b) tungsten has a high atomic number and a high melting point.
c) characteristic radiation is independent of the atomic number of the target.
d) most characteristic radiation relates to outer electron shell vacancies.
e) larger focal spots have greater local heat loading than smaller.

29 In radio-isotope studies of the urinary tract

a) acute urinary tract infection is a contraindication.
b) Tc99m DTPA is cleared by glomerular filtration.
c) captopril is used in assessment of renovascular hypertension.
d) Tc99m mercaptoacetyltriglycine (MAG-3) is the best agent for assessment of renal cortical scarring.
e) micturating cystography is less sensitive than the conventional radiographic technique for reflux.

30 The air gap technique

a) decreases scatter by means of filtration.
b) decreases patient exposure.
c) usually requires less exposure than with the use of a grid.
d) results in a magnified image.
e) when used in chest radiography the focus-film distance is increased to ten feet.

31 In the pelvis and hips

a) on an AP view the lesser trochanter is obscured on medial rotation of the hip.
b) the femoral neck is elongated on an AP view of the hip in lateral rotation.
c) heels should be close together for an AP view of both hips.
d) the centring point for an AP view of both hips is 2·5cms above the pubic symphysis.
e) the superior pubic ramus overlies the acetabulum on a properly positioned lateral hip view.

32 In generator design

a) single phase generators have highest voltage ripple.
b) increased voltage ripple leads to higher patient radiation dose.
c) three phase generators give a higher tube output for a given tube current.
d) three phase generators have slow exposure time control.
e) high frequency invertor generators have very small voltage ripple.

33 In geometry of the radiographic image

a) magnification is the ratio of focus-film to focus-object distances.
b) the penumbra is independent of focal spot size.
c) the penumbra is narrower on the anode side.
d) position relative to the centre of the beam has no effect.
e) the penumbra is not affected by distance from the focus.

34 In Doppler ultrasound

a) a single piezoelectric crystal is used in pulsed Doppler.
b) the usual frequency used is from 3 to 8Mhz.
c) the Doppler shift is independent of incident angle.
d) the intensity of the scattered beam is proportional to the square of the frequency.
e) the maximum detectable Doppler shift equals half the pulse repetition frequency.

35 In MRI of the abdomen

a) oral contrast agents may increase or decrease the signal.
b) the T1 and T2 of liver are shorter than those of spleen.
c) intrahepatic ducts can not be clearly seen.
d) the hepatic vasculature is poorly defined.
e) surface coils are necessary to show a normal pancreatic duct.

36 In the pelvis and lower limb

a) the obturator foramen lies below Shenton's line.
b) a lateral view of the hip shows the ipsilateral obturator foramen well.
c) free fat in the knee is best seen on a skyline projection.
d) the os trigonum is most closely related to the calcaneum.
e) the calcaneum articulates distally with the cuboid.

37 The following are true of image intensifiers

a) the conversion factor relates output luminance to input exposure rate.
b) the minification gain is the ratio of input to output phosphor diameters.
c) the flux gain increases the brightness by a factor of approximately 50.
d) the brightness gain is unrelated to its age.
e) a uniform image is produced.

38 In the pharynx

a) the opening of the Eustachian tube lies below and in front of the pharyngeal recess.
b) the lower border is the inferior aspect of the cricoid cartilage.
c) the piriform fossae extend outside the thyrohyoid membrane.
d) cricopharyngeus forms the sphincteric part of the inferior constrictor muscle.
e) the middle constrictor muscle arises from the hyoid bone.

39 Within the brain

a) the thalamus lies medial to the internal capsule.
b) the external capsule lies medial to the putamen.
c) the corticospinal tract passes through the posterior limb of the internal capsule.
d) the basal nuclei are composed of white matter.
e) the claustrum lies lateral to the external capsule.

40 Conventional (ionic) water soluble contrast media

a) have an osmolarity up to eight times that of plasma.
b) cause histamine release from mast cells.
c) containing meglumine only are less cardiotoxic than a sodium/meglumine mixture.
d) containing meglumine are more neurotoxic than those containing sodium.
e) containing sodium salts are more toxic to vascular endothelium than meglumine salts.

41 In MRI sequences

a) TR refers to the time between the start of two sequential 90° pulses.
b) TE refers to the time from the start of the 90° pulse to the start of the echo.
c) a T1 weighted image uses a short TR and a short TE.
d) a T2 weighted image uses a short TR and a long TE.
e) proton density images are obtained using a long TR and a short TE.

42 The formation of a latent image involves

a) the presence of point defects in the lattice.
b) the use of allylthiourea to create sensitivity specks.
c) a minimum of two silver atoms to create an image.
d) both the photoelectric and Compton effects.
e) deposition of bromine atoms in the latent image centre.

43 Regarding the facial bones

a) the base line is at 45° to the central ray for an occipitomental (OM) view.
b) the zygomatic arches are seen better on an OM than an OM30 projection.
c) a lateral view should use a horizontal beam in trauma cases.
d) the median sagittal plane is perpendicular to the film for a lateral view.
e) the 30° caudal fronto-occipital projection demonstrates the zygomatic arches.

44 The pineal gland

a) lies between the superior colliculi.
b) is directly inferior to the splenium of the corpus callosum.
c) stalk is divided by the third ventricle into superior and inferior laminae.
d) receives blood supply from the middle cerebral arteries.
e) lies within 3mms of the midline.

45 The following are true of the pancreas

a) the uncinate process lies behind the superior mesenteric vessels.
b) the inferior vena cava lies directly behind the pancreatic head.
c) the common bile duct runs in the anterior aspect of the head.
d) the posterior surface is related to the splenic vein.
e) the pancreatic duct lies in the anterior half.

46 In estimating the gestational age of the foetus

a) the gestational sac is visible transvaginally at three menstrual weeks.
b) the crown-rump length is a suitable method up to 16 weeks.
c) the biparietal diameter is more accurate in early than late pregnancy.
d) the biparietal diameter should be measured at the level of the thalami.
e) femur length is most accurate close to term.

47 In urinary tract intervention

a) cyst puncture is contraindicated if hydatid disease is suspected.
b) vesico-ureteric reflux should be excluded prior to renal pressure studies.
c) normal renal pressure should be approximately 20cms of water at an infusion rate of 10mls/min.
d) ureteric fistula is a contraindication to percutaneous nephrostomy.
e) haemolysis is a complication of percutaneous nephrolithotomy.

48 Regarding submandibular sialography

a) Wharton's duct opens beside the frenulum.
b) suitable control films include an inferosuperior (occlusal) view.
c) up to 2mls of contrast medium is used normally.
d) it is normal to see residual contrast medium in the ducts post emptying.
e) there are no contraindications to the procedure.

49 In examination of the small bowel

a) glucagon interferes with transit time.
b) flocculation of barium occurs frequently during a small bowel enema.
c) prone films separate bowel loops.
d) transit time for barium is reduced by adding Gastrografin.
e) metoclopramide is contraindicated.

50 In the abdomen

a) a plain abdominal radiograph requires a high mA and a short time exposure.
b) an erect abdominal radiograph requires a lower kV than a supine one.
c) a left lateral decubitus view is preferred to a right lateral.
d) the beam is tilted 15° caudally for an AP view of the urinary bladder.
e) in the prone position the lowest point of the gallbladder is the neck.

51 In magnetic resonance imaging

a) only nuclei with odd numbers of neutrons or protons are suitable for imaging.
b) most carbon atoms are detectable.
c) hydrogen content differs in normal and diseased tissue.
d) hydrogen nuclei are randomly oriented when no external magnetic field is applied.
e) external magnetic field causes net magnetisation of hydrogen transverse to the field.

52 In the thorax

a) the second rib articulates with the sternum at the manubriosternal junction.
b) a sternal foramen is a normal variant.
c) the subclavian artery is the most lateral vessel crossing the first rib.
d) the costal cartilages have no muscular or ligamentous attachments.
e) the subclavian vessels lie inferior to a long cervical rib, when present.

53 Regarding patient protection

a) gonad shields should always be used.
b) patient dose can be decreased by the use of carbon fibre tables.
c) total beam filtration should never be less than 0·5mm aluminium equivalent.
d) radiography of areas remote from a foetus can be safely performed at any stage during pregnancy.
e) the direction of a beam has no effect on dose delivered.

54 The following are true of magnets used in MRI

a) superconducting magnets operate at 4° Celsius.
b) typical strengths range from 0·5 to 1·5 Tesla.
c) they require cooling by hydrogen.
d) superconducting magnets have more homogenous magnetic fields than resistive types.
e) resistive magnets create large amounts of heat.

55 In stereoradiography

a) lateral tube movement is about 10% of focus-film distance.
b) greater tube shift allows greater depth appreciation.
c) grid use limits the amount of tube shift.
d) an alternative method is to shift the patient slightly for each exposure.
e) viewing of the stereoradiographs is critical for success.

56 Knee arthrography

a) requires up to 40mls of air for double contrast studies.
b) cannot be performed in the presence of a total knee replacement.
c) involves siting the needle 1 to 2cms posterior to the lower pole of the patella.
d) demonstrates the menisci best on prone spot films.
e) delayed films can aid visualisation of loose bodies.

57 In radiography of the foot and ankle

a) the dorsiplantar (AP) view of the foot is centred to the cuboid-navicular joint.
b) oblique views of the foot require the foot to be tilted to more than 60 degrees.
c) the subtalar joints are best seen in the oblique position.
d) an AP view of the ankle is taken in lateral rotation.
e) stress views of the ankle are performed routinely by the radiographer.

58 In the production of x-rays

a) bremsstrahlung radiation occurs due to interactions with nuclei.
b) characteristic radiation occurs due to interaction with inner electrons.
c) characteristic radiation for a tungsten target occurs at 60kV.
d) the continuous spectrum is dependent on the voltage.
e) bremsstrahlung radiation is more important than characteristic radiation in mammography tubes.

59 In magnetic resonance angiography

a) 2D time of flight studies are only useful for vessels with a high flow rate.
b) 3D time of flight studies have better resolution than 2D.
c) phase contrast angiography eliminates signal from high intensity stationary material.
d) flow compensation methods take account of a wide range of velocities.
e) phase contrast angiograms are adversely affected by magnetisation saturation.

60 Intensifying screens

a) do not affect resolution.
b) help reduce patient dose.
c) may increase noise on the final image.
d) have phosphorescent properties.
e) absorb more photons when the thickness is increased.

Paper One

Answers

Paper One   Answers

1.
- a) T
- b) T
- c) F — several.
- d) F — external carotid.
- e) T

Gray's Anatomy, 38th Ed., 1995, Ch.10.

2.
- a) T
- b) T
- c) T
- d) T
- e) F — inferior mesenteric artery.

Gray's Anatomy, 38th Ed., 1995, Ch.3.

3.
- a) T
- b) T — axillary tail of Spence.
- c) T — Astley Cooper ligaments.
- d) T
- e) F — additional supply from the second to fourth intercostal arteries.

Gray's Anatomy, 38th Ed., 1995, Ch.5.

4.
- a) T
- b) F — more dilute for bile ducts.
- c) T
- d) F
- e) T

A Guide to Radiological Procedures, Chapman & Nakielny, 3rd Ed., 1993, Ch.4.
A Textbook of Radiology and Imaging, Sutton, 5th Ed., 1993, Ch.33.

5.
- a) F
- b) T — to assess discs above or below.
- c) F — irritant; confuse interpretation of provoked pain.
- d) T — more if disc is damaged.
- e) F — less.

A Guide to Radiological Procedures, Chapman & Nakielny, 3rd Ed., 1993, Ch.12.

Paper One   Answers

6
- a) F
- b) F
- c) F   especially if a tourniquet is used.
- d) T   as it bypasses the axillary vein.
- e) T

A Guide to Radiological Procedures, Chapman & Nakielny, 3rd Ed., 1993, Ch.9.

7
- a) F   to halve intensity.
- b) F   per centimetre, i.e. 1/cm.
- c) T
- d) F   sum.
- e) F   monochromatic only.

Christensen's Physics of Diagnostic Radiology, Curry et al, 4th Ed., 1990, Ch.5.

8
- a) F   also ophthalmic artery.
- b) T
- c) T   and becomes the infra-orbital nerve.
- d) F   turns backwards.
- e) F   at arch of aorta on left; at subclavian level on right.

Gray's Anatomy, 38th Ed., 1995, Ch.8.

9
- a) T
- b) F   thicker posteriorly.
- c) F   corniculate and cuneiform are also fibro-elastic cartilage.
- d) T
- e) T

Gray's Anatomy, 38th Ed., 1995, Ch.11.

10
- a) T
- b) T
- c) F   50%.
- d) T
- e) T

Practical Nuclear Medicine, Sharp et al, 1989, Ch.19.

Paper One   Answers

11 a) T
    b) F   vas above seminal vesicles.
    c) F   vesico-uterine pouch, not pouch of Douglas.
    d) F   the median umbilical ligament - urachal remnant.
    e) T

Gray's Anatomy, 38th Ed., 1995, Ch.13.

12 a) T
    b) T
    c) F   pons.
    d) F   fourth ventricle.
    e) T

Gray's Anatomy, 38th Ed., 1995, Ch.8.

13 a) T
    b) T
    c) F   free electron is not under the influence of the nucleus.
    d) T   energy equals the difference between the two shells involved.
    e) F   more likely to be chemically reactive and magnetic.

Radiographics, 1997, 17, 967-984.

14 a) F   tail.
    b) T
    c) T
    d) T
    e) T

Gray's Anatomy, 38th Ed., 1995, Ch.14.

15 a) T
    b) T
    c) T   absorbs light transmitted through the base.
    d) T
    e) F   reducing latitude increases contrast.

Radiographics, 1996, 16, 1467-1479.

Paper One   Answers

16 a) F   recess of greater sac.
    b) F   inferior border.
    c) T
    d) T
    e) T

Gray's Anatomy, 38th Ed., 1995, Ch.9.

17 a) F   glucoheptonate has faster plasma clearance.
    b) T   needs prior blocking with potassium perchlorate.
    c) F   hence uptake in abnormal tissue.
    d) T   similar to glucoheptonate.
    e) F   can improve sensitivity.

A Guide to Radiological Procedures, Chapman & Nakielny, 3rd Ed., 1993, Ch.12.

18 a) F   70%.
    b) T
    c) T   common hepatic.
    d) F   behind.
    e) T   collaterals in disease of the common iliac vessels.

An Atlas of Radiological Anatomy, Weir & Abrahams, 2nd Ed., 1986.

19 a) T
    b) F
    c) T
    d) F
    e) T

An Atlas of Radiological Anatomy, Weir & Abrahams, 2nd Ed., 1986.

20 a) T
    b) T
    c) F   full general anaesthetic.
    d) F   after three months progressive ossification makes examination difficult.
    e) T

Techniques in Diagnostic Imaging, Whitehouse et al, 2nd Ed., 1990, Ch.24.

Paper One   Answers

21 a) T
    b) T
    c) F   superficial.
    d) T
    e) F

Gray's Anatomy, 38th Ed., 1995, Ch.10.

22 a) T
    b) F
    c) F   sodium iodide.
    d) T
    e) F   less than parallel collimator; best suited for small parts.

Radiographics, 1996, 16, 173-183.

23 a) T
    b) F   inferolateral, for coracoclavicular ligament.
    c) F   anatomical neck is immediately distal to the head.
    d) T
    e) F

Gray's Anatomy, 38th Ed., 1995, Ch.6.

24 a) T
    b) F
    c) T
    d) T
    e) F

Gray's Anatomy, 38th Ed., 1995, Ch.7.

25 a) F   150 to 180cms; 300cms for air gap technique.
    b) F
    c) F   cranial.
    d) T
    e) T

Clark's Positioning in Radiography, Swallow et al, 11th Ed., 1986, Ch.13.
Making the best use of a Department of Clinical Radiology; Royal College of Radiologists London, 2nd Ed., 1993.

Paper One   Answers

26 a) F
    b) F
    c) T
    d) T
    e) F

Gray's Anatomy, 38th Ed., 1995, Ch.12.

27 a) T   but not solely; also radiation exposure, recording system characteristics.
    b) F
    c) F   usually detrimental to image quality.
    d) T
    e) T

Radiographics, 1997, 17, 479-498.

28 a) F   tube current very sensitive to change in filament current.
    b) T
    c) F
    d) F   innermost, K-shell vacancies.
    e) F

Radiographics, 1997, 17, 1259-1268.

29 a) F
    b) T
    c) T
    d) F   Tc99m dimercaptosuccinic acid (DMSA).
    e) F   at least as sensitive.

A Guide to Radiological Procedures, Chapman & Nakielny, 3rd Ed., 1993, Ch.5.

30 a) F   scatter misses the film.
    b) F
    c) T
    d) T   because of the increased focus-film distance.
    e) T

Christensen's Physics of Diagnostic Radiology, Curry et al, 4th Ed., 1990, Ch.8.

Paper One   Answers

---

31 a) T
b) F   foreshortened.
c) F   heels separated, legs medially rotated.
d) T
e) F   this occurs when patient is tilted too much to the side in question.

Clark's Positioning in Radiography, Swallow et al, 11th Ed., 1986, Ch.4.

32 a) T
b) T   slightly higher.
c) T
d) F   very fast.
e) T

Radiographics, 1997, 17, 1533-1557.

33 a) T
b) F
c) T
d) F
e) F

Christensen's Physics of Diagnostic Radiology, Curry et al, 4th Ed., 1990, Ch.15.

34 a) T
b) T
c) F
d) F   frequency to the fourth power.
e) T

Christensen's Physics of Diagnostic Radiology, Curry et al, 4th Ed., 1990, Ch.20.

35 a) T
b) T
c) F
d) F
e) T

A Textbook of Radiology and Imaging, Sutton, 5th Ed., 1993, Chs.34,35.
A Textbook of Radiology and Imaging, Sutton, 6th Ed., 1997, Chs.34,35.

Paper One   Answers

36 a) T medial part of the line is the inferior aspect of the superior pubic ramus.
    b) F
    c) F horizontal beam lateral view.
    d) F talus.
    e) T

An Atlas of Radiological Anatomy, Weir & Abrahams, 2nd Ed., 1986.

37 a) T
    b) F the square of this ratio.
    c) T
    d) F
    e) F vignetting and peripheral distortion occur.

Christensen's Physics of Diagnostic Radiology, Curry et al, 4th Ed., 1990, Ch.12.

38 a) T
    b) T
    c) F lateral boundaries are the thyroid cartilage and thyrohyoid membrane.
    d) T thyropharyngeus forms the propulsion part.
    e) T

Gray's Anatomy, 38th Ed., 1995, Ch.12.

39 a) T posterior limb.
    b) F lateral.
    c) T
    d) F grey matter.
    e) T medial to the Sylvian fissure.

Gray's Anatomy, 38th Ed., 1995, Ch.8.

40 a) T
    b) T
    c) F mixture less toxic than either alone.
    d) F
    e) T

Techniques in Diagnostic Imaging, Whitehouse et al, 2nd Ed., 1990, Ch.30.

Paper One   Answers

---

41 a) T   i.e., time to repeat
    b) F   time from end of 90° pulse to start of echo.
    c) T
    d) F   long TR and long TE.
    e) T

MRI made easy, Schild, 1990.

42 a) T
    b) T
    c) T
    d) T
    e) F   bromine migrates into gelatin.

Christensen's Physics of Diagnostic Radiology, Curry et al, 4th Ed., 1990, Ch.10.

43 a) T
    b) F
    c) T   to show fluid levels in sinuses.
    d) F   parallel.
    e) T   best seen if film is underpenetrated.

Clark's Positioning in Radiography, Swallow et al, 11th Ed., 1986, Ch.10.

44 a) T
    b) F   separated from it by tela choroidea of third ventricle and contained veins.
    c) T
    d) F   posterior cerebral via posterior choroidal arteries.
    e) T

Gray's Anatomy, 38th Ed., 1995, Ch.15.
A Textbook of Radiology and Imaging, Sutton, 5th Ed., 1993, Ch.53.

45 a) T
    b) T
    c) F   posterior, or within it.
    d) T
    e) F   slightly posterior.

Gray's Anatomy, 38th Ed., 1995, Ch.12.

Paper One   Answers

46
- a) **F** five weeks.
- b) **F** best between seven and nine weeks transvaginally.
- c) **T**
- d) **T**
- e) **F** best early second trimester.

Ultrasonography in Obstetrics and Gynecology, Callen, 3rd Ed., 1994, Ch.7.

47
- a) **T**
- b) **T**
- c) **F** no greater than 13cms water; 20 or more indicates obstruction.
- d) **F** may allow fistula to close.
- e) **T** due to irrigating fluid.

A Guide to Radiological Procedures, Chapman & Nakielny, 3rd Ed., 1993, Ch.5.

48
- a) **T**
- b) **T**
- c) **T**
- d) **F**
- e) **F**

A Textbook of Radiology and Imaging, Sutton, 6th Ed., 1997, Ch.28.
A Guide to Radiological Procedures, Chapman & Nakielny, 3rd Ed., 1993, Ch.14.

49
- a) **F** unlike Buscopan.
- b) **F** unlikely due to rapid passage.
- c) **T**
- d) **T**
- e) **F**

A Guide to Radiological Procedures, Chapman & Nakielny, 3rd Ed., 1993, Ch.3.

50
- a) **T**
- b) **F** slightly higher kV.
- c) **T** gas rises above liver.
- d) **T**
- e) **F** fundus.

Clark's Positioning in Radiography, Swallow et al, 11th Ed., 1986, Ch.14.

Paper One   Answers

---

51 a) T   even numbers pair off and cancel each other out.
    b) F   only C_{13}, which is 1·1% of atomic carbon.
    c) T   due to different water content.
    d) T
    e) F   along direction of field, a lower energy state.

Radiographics, 1994, 14, 829-846.

52 a) T
    b) T   due to incomplete fusion.
    c) F   medial to subclavian vein.
    d) F   have partial attachments of anterior abdominal muscles.
    e) F   superior.

Gray's Anatomy, 38th Ed., 1995, Ch.6.

53 a) F   not if it interferes with the diagnostic image.
    b) T
    c) T
    d) T   with appropriate collimation and shielding.
    e) F   PA beam decreases dose to breast, lens etc..

Guidance Notes For The Protection of Persons Against Ionising Radiation Arising From Medical and Dental Use, National Radiation Protection Board, 1988.

54 a) F   4°Kelvin (-269°Celsius).
    b) T
    c) F   helium, nitrogen.
    d) T
    e) T   which must be dissipated.

MRI made easy, Schild, 1990.

55 a) T   5 to 15%.
    b) T
    c) T
    d) F
    e) T   each eye must see the corresponding shifted image.

Clark's Positioning in Radiography, Swallow et al, 11th Ed., 1986, Ch.21.

Paper One   Answers

---

56   a)   T
      b)   F
      c)   F
      d)   T
      e)   T

A Guide to Radiological Procedures, Chapman & Nakielny, 3rd Ed., 1993, Ch.11.

57   a)   T
      b)   F   30 to 45 degrees.
      c)   T
      d)   F   medially with dorsiflexion.
      e)   F

Clark's Positioning in Radiography, Swallow et al, 11th Ed., 1986, Ch.3.

58   a)   T
      b)   T
      c)   F   70kV.
      d)   T
      e)   F

Christensen's Physics of Diagnostic Radiology, Curry et al, 4th Ed., 1990, Ch.2.

59   a)   F   sensitive to slow flow; can distinguish slow flow and occlusions.
      b)   T   useful for tortuous vessels.
      c)   T   these can mimic flow signal in time of flight studies.
      d)   F   take account of constant velocity; may overestimate stenoses.
      e)   F   this helps avoid problems.

Radiographics, 1995, 15, 453-465.

60   a)   F   some degree of resolution is lost.
      b)   T
      c)   T
      d)   F   fluorescent; phosphorescence is delayed emission of light.
      e)   T

Radiographics, 1996, 16, 903-916.

Paper Two

Questions

Paper Two Questions

1 In skull radiography

   a) the median sagittal plane and the interorbital line are perpendicular to the film for a lateral view.
   b) occipito-frontal 20 views are taken with the beam angled cranially to the base-line.
   c) Towne's views are taken with the orbito-meatal line and median sagittal plane perpendicular to the film.
   d) the submentovertical view is the projection of choice for the skull base.
   e) the optic foramina are best radiographed in the supine oblique position.

2 The following are true of radiographic contrast

   a) low kVp technique yields high contrast.
   b) high kVp technique allows a greater exposure latitude.
   c) the mAs used affects both density and contrast.
   d) film blackening is indirectly proportional to kVp.
   e) fog reduces contrast due to increased film density.

3 Regarding the extraperitoneal spaces in the abdomen

   a) the anterior pararenal space is confined laterally by the lateroconal fascia.
   b) fat in the posterior pararenal space forms the 'flank stripe'.
   c) the adrenal glands lie in the posterior pararenal space.
   d) the perirenal spaces are not usually continuous across the midline.
   e) the ascending colon lies in the posterior pararenal space.

4 In the gastrointestinal tract

   a) oily contrast medium may be used for sialography.
   b) the upper oesophagus is narrowest at the cricoid cartilage level.
   c) the duodenum is completely covered with peritoneum.
   d) the maximum diameter of the normal jejunum is 5cms.
   e) lactose should be added to barium to diagnose disaccharidase deficiency.

5 The following are true of a CT image

   a) the image is usually reconstructed by simple back projection methods.
   b) the Hounsfield unit determines the attenuation relative to water.
   c) the window level refers to the average Hounsfield unit displayed.
   d) the window width refers to the range of Hounsfield units displayed.
   e) noise values must vary by more than 2 to 4 Hounsfield units to be significant.

Paper Two   Questions

6   Regarding water soluble oral contrast media

a) Gastrografin is ionic.
b) Gastrografin is safe to use in cases of suspected aspiration.
c) Gastromiro has a similar side effect profile to Gastrografin.
d) their use is safe in suspected perforation.
e) they may be both diagnostic and therapeutic.

7   Regarding the heart

a) the aortic valve usually has two cusps.
b) on a PA chest x-ray the mitral valve lies at a higher level than the tricuspid.
c) the aortic valve lies below the pulmonary valve on a PA chest x-ray.
d) the ductus arteriosus carries blood from the pulmonary artery to the aorta in the foetus.
e) the foramen ovale connects the right and left ventricles.

8   Beam hardening

a) involves selective removal of lower energy x-rays.
b) decreases the average energy of the beam.
c) causes a more mono-energetic beam.
d) lowers the maximum energy of an x-ray spectrum.
e) is of no use in mammography.

9   In scatter

a) total absorption of a photon is due to the photoelectric effect.
b) Compton scatter is independent of photon energy.
c) Compton scatter does not affect image contrast.
d) an air gap is most effective at higher energies.
e) an air gap causes photons to miss the image receptor.

10   The following are true of dose limits for members of the public

a) the whole body limit is 5 milliSieverts (0·5 rems) per annum.
b) the lens should receive less than 30 milliSieverts (3 rems) per annum.
c) the dose limit to the skin is 50 milliSieverts (5 rems) per annum.
d) the extremities should receive less than 50 milliSieverts (5 rems) per annum.
e) these limits apply to patients as members of the public.

Paper Two   Questions

11   Sources of increased radiographic noise include

a) quantum mottle.
b) film grain.
c) film processing artefacts.
d) x-ray to light conversion.
e) high x-ray exposure.

12   In the femur

a) the lesser trochanter lies on the anteromedial aspect of the upper femur.
b) the fovea gives attachment to the ligament of the head of the femur.
c) the anterior surface of the femoral neck is entirely intracapsular.
d) the posterior surface of the femoral neck is entirely intracapsular.
e) the lateral femoral condyle has a smaller patellar surface than the medial.

13   In breast studies

a) mammography tubes use a molybdenum target and filter.
b) the standard views are craniocaudal and lateral oblique.
c) a single view mammogram gives an average dose of 2 milliGrays.
d) xeroradiography causes edge enhancement.
e) galactography is used to investigate nipple discharge.

14   For oesophageal swallow examination

a) barium is the most suitable agent to show a perforation.
b) the erect position is best for identifying varices.
c) a non-ionic agent is preferred for diagnosis of tracheo-oesophageal fistula in children.
d) barium is contraindicated if a web is suspected.
e) the patient should be in the right posterior oblique position.

15   In cerebral angiography

a) visualisation of the thalamostriate vein allows assessment of the size of the lateral ventricle.
b) the capillary phase is clearly distinguished from arterial and venous phases.
c) the anterior choroidal artery is variable in position.
d) the venous angle is visible in almost all examinations and is constant.
e) the posterior fossa veins are constant in position.

16 In the ear

a) the malleus is the most lateral of the ossicles.
b) the pharyngotympanic tube (Eustachian/auditory) connects the nasopharynx and the inner ear.
c) the ossicles connect the tympanic membrane and cochlea.
d) the tegmen tympani is a thick bony plate between the tympanic and cranial cavities.
e) the stapes attaches to the round window.

17 In the eye

a) the eyeball is smaller in women than men.
b) the choroid layer is avascular.
c) the choroid is loosely attached to the retina.
d) the retina is thickest near the optic disc.
e) the retina is thickest at the fovea.

18 In magnetic resonance equipment

a) magnetic field gradients encode position within the imaged volume.
b) resistive magnets require helium for cooling.
c) low field strength magnets have higher signal to noise ratio than high field strengths.
d) shimming improves the uniformity of the magnetic field.
e) chemical shift occurs at fat-water interfaces.

19 In Doppler ultrasound

a) continuous wave Doppler has good depth resolution.
b) continuous wave Doppler is more sensitive than pulsed Doppler.
c) the Doppler effect is lost perpendicular to the flow.
d) motion towards the transducer gives a higher frequency Doppler shift.
e) aliasing is a problem with continuous wave Doppler.

20 Within the skull

a) the dura mater is composed of a single dense layer.
b) the inferior sagittal sinus runs in the free lower edge of the falx cerebri.
c) the superior petrosal sinuses lie in the tentorium cerebelli.
d) the tentorium is attached to the anterior clinoid processes.
e) the dura mater remains separate from the pia and arachnoid mater in the sella turcica.

21 Lymphangiography

a) can not detect tumour in normal sized glands.
b) is technically easy to perform.
c) allows surveillance of glands over time.
d) is poor at assessing internal iliac nodes.
e) reduces pulmonary ventilatory function.

22 Regarding upper gastrointestinal studies in children

a) the supine position is preferred for assessment of tracheo-oesophageal fistulae.
b) when examining for tracheo-oesophageal fistulae, less than 5mls of contrast medium is adequate.
c) 10mls of low density barium is suitable for diagnosis of a hiatus hernia.
d) pyloric stenosis is best diagnosed by ultrasound in fasting infants.
e) suspected malrotation may be diagnosed by ultrasound.

23 In quality control of film processing

a) intensifying screen output changes with time.
b) film characteristics remain constant long after expiry date.
c) developer pH and specific gravity should be measured.
d) photographic chemicals oxidise over time if they are not used.
e) bulk buying of films and chemicals is helpful.

24 In radiography of the hand

a) the PA view centres to the head of the third metacarpal.
b) abduction demonstrates the scaphoid more clearly.
c) single views are adequate for the phalanges.
d) the definition of a PA thumb view is unaffected by the increased object-film distance.
e) a ball-catcher's view is a supplementary view used to improve visualisation of joints.

25 Protons

a) are normally evenly distributed in parallel and anti-parallel directions.
b) precess in equal and opposite directions.
c) have a Larmor frequency proportional to the external magnetic field.
d) have a gyromagnetic ratio of 42·5MHz/Tesla.
e) produce a net longitudinal magnetisation which can be directly measured.

Paper Two   Questions

26   In the shoulder region

   a)   an AP view should be taken erect in suspected shoulder dislocation.
   b)   supraspinatus inserts low on the greater tuberosity of the humerus.
   c)   cranial angulation of the beam facilitates demonstration of tendon calcification.
   d)   acromioclavicular joints should be examined with a single exposure AP view.
   e)   25° cranial angulation of the central ray is required for the acromioclavicular joints.

27   In the pelvis

   a)   the pelvic diaphragm is formed by levator ani and coccygeus.
   b)   levator ani forms the medial boundary of the ischiorectal fossa.
   c)   the internal pudendal vessels lie in the roof of the ischiorectal fossa.
   d)   the obturator canal lies in the inferior margin of the obturator membrane.
   e)   the sciatic nerve emerges above piriformis.

28   Regarding the kidneys

   a)   they lie anterior to the arcuate ligaments of the diaphragm.
   b)   the right kidney is related anteriorly to the second part of the duodenum.
   c)   the left kidney is related anteriorly to loops of jejunum.
   d)   the anterior pararenal space is limited posteriorly by the anterior layer of the renal fascia.
   e)   the posterior pararenal space is limited posteriorly by transversalis fascia.

29   In film processing

   a)   developer reduces exposed silver halide to its metallic form.
   b)   developers are alkaline solutions.
   c)   developers act at high pH.
   d)   organic antifoggants are included in developer.
   e)   fixers stop development by increasing pH.

30   In the brain

   a)   the anterior cerebral vessels lie on the corpus callosum.
   b)   the corpus callosum forms the roof of the lateral ventricle.
   c)   the inferior sagittal sinus lies on the splenium of the corpus callosum.
   d)   the corpus callosum is always present.
   e)   the septum pellucidum is formed from a single lamina of grey and white matter.

31 In the abdomen and pelvis

a) the left renal vein lies between the aorta and superior mesenteric artery.
b) the superior mesenteric vein lies to the right of the superior mesenteric artery.
c) the right common iliac artery crosses the left common iliac vein.
d) the left common iliac artery crosses the right common iliac vein.
e) the vesical arteries arise from the external iliac artery.

32 The following are true of grids

a) their use decreases patient dose.
b) the grid ratio relates the height to the width of the lead strips.
c) the lead strips are approximately 0·05mm thick.
d) the Bucky factor is the ratio of incident to transmitted radiation.
e) the contrast improvement factor (K) is the ratio of the radiographic contrast with a grid to that without a grid.

33 Regarding the lungs

a) the oblique fissures arise at the level of T4/5 and run through both hila.
b) the azygos fissure contains four layers of pleura and is visible in less than 1% of the population.
c) the superior accessory fissure separates the apical and basal segments of the lower lobe.
d) the azygos vein runs inferior to the right hilum.
e) the phrenic nerves run posterior to both hila.

34 The filament of an x-ray tube

a) is usually made of tungsten.
b) is heated by a current of 3 to 5 milliamperes.
c) has maximum thermionic emission at 1500° Celsius.
d) lies in a focusing cup which is usually at the same negative potential.
e) when double, both filaments are used for large exposures.

35 A caesium iodide input phosphor in an image intensifier

a) has randomly oriented crystals.
b) has a greater packing density than zinc cadmium sulphide.
c) is typically 0·1mm thick.
d) yields resolution of three to five line pairs per centimetre.
e) will absorb approximately two-thirds of the incident beam.

36 The parathyroid glands

a) derive from the third and fourth pharyngeal pouches.
b) lie external to the thyroid capsule.
c) receive blood supply from the inferior thyroid artery.
d) are all constant in position.
e) are closely related to the recurrent laryngeal nerve.

37 In radionuclide imaging of the thyroid and parathyroids

a) technetium99m pertechnetate is organified in a similar fashion to iodine.
b) iodine 123 is suitable for use.
c) technetium99m pertechnetate is the best agent for visualisation of a retrosternal goitre.
d) technetium/thallium subtraction imaging is used to identify thyroid tissue.
e) technetium studies of the thyroid give an effective dose of 1 milliSievert.

38 Regarding radiopharmaceuticals

a) their half life should be as short as possible.
b) they should be gamma ray emitters in the energy range 50 to 300kV.
c) the effective half life is proportional to the product of the physical and biological half lives.
d) a technetium99m photon has an energy emission of 0·14meV.
e) the most commonly used radionuclides are produced in a cyclotron.

39 The following are suitable contrast media for myelography

a) carbon dioxide.
b) lipiodol.
c) iopamidol.
d) iotrolan.
e) myodil.

40 In soft tissue radiography

a) a high kVp is used in xeroradiography.
b) low kVp should be used to detect surgical emphysema.
c) calcification is usually best demonstrated by low kVp technique.
d) talc and deodorant cause artefacts on mammograms.
e) 1mm focal spot tubes are advised for mammography.

41 In the physics of x-ray production

a) α-particles have a single unit of positive charge.
b) electromagnetic radiation can travel in a vacuum.
c) the frequency of electromagnetic radiation is inversely related to its wavelength.
d) an x-ray and γ-ray of the same energy are indistinguishable.
e) stationary charged particles are affected by magnetic fields.

42 Regarding calcium tungstate screens

a) they have an intrinsic conversion efficiency of approximately 5%.
b) the screen efficiency is approximately 50%.
c) the intensification factor is the ratio of the exposures needed to produce the same film density with and without the screen.
d) higher speed produces finer detail.
e) the presence of dye in the phosphor layer decreases screen speed.

43 In the venous system

a) the long saphenous vein is the major vein of the deep system of the leg.
b) the deep dorsal vein of the penis drains into the prostatic venous plexus.
c) the inferior vena cava is in direct contact with the right ureter.
d) the left testicular vein enters the anterior aspect of the inferior vena cava.
e) the splenic vein drains the pancreas.

44 Regarding the intestine

a) the cardiac notch separates the left border of the oesophagus from the gastric fundus.
b) the gastric vessels lie along the greater curvature of the stomach.
c) the stomach contains three muscle layers.
d) the duodenum turns abruptly backwards at the duodenojejunal flexure.
e) the first part of the duodenum is closely related to the gallbladder.

45 Around the knee joint

a) the adductor canal lies deep to sartorius, on adductor longus.
b) gracilis is separated from the tibial collateral ligament by a bursa.
c) there is a single aponeurotic opening in adductor magnus.
d) the tendon of popliteus is extracapsular.
e) the suprapatellar bursa develops separately from the knee joint.

Paper Two   Questions

46   Compton scatter is

    a)   inversely proportional to energy.
    b)   proportional to atomic number.
    c)   predominantly forwards at diagnostic kVs.
    d)   not a safety hazard.
    e)   due to interaction of photons with free electrons.

47   Regarding the paranasal sinuses

    a)   the frontal sinuses may be absent at birth.
    b)   the ethmoid sinuses are separated from the orbit by a thick plate of bone.
    c)   the sphenoid sinuses are related to the optic chiasm.
    d)   the sphenoid sinuses open into the superior meatus.
    e)   the maxillary antrum is related to the upper molars and the second upper premolar.

48   In the upper limb

    a)   the coracoid process is clearly seen on an axial view of the shoulder.
    b)   the lesser tuberosity of the humerus is seen in profile on an AP view of the shoulder.
    c)   the radial tuberosity lies directly against the ulna on an AP view of the elbow.
    d)   the distal radius articulates with the triquetrum.
    e)   views in ulnar deviation show the scaphoid well.

49   A lateral view of the skull will show

    a)   habenular calcification.
    b)   adenoidal soft tissue.
    c)   the foramen lacerum.
    d)   the internal auditory canals.
    e)   the lambdoid sutures.

50   The following are true of the uterus

    a)   the cervix is the inferior limit of the pouch of Douglas.
    b)   it lies completely below the pelvic inlet.
    c)   retroversion is defined as posterior inclination of the uterus so that the cervix faces forwards.
    d)   the uterine artery supplies the lateral two-thirds of the fallopian tube.
    e)   the round ligament attaches to the pelvic side wall.

51 Regarding tomographic technique

a) autotomography has no practical applications.
b) tomography of the larynx is performed with the patient phonating.
c) linear movement is the best form of tomography for imaging the bronchi and lungs.
d) renal tomography has a typical fulcrum of 8 to 11cms.
e) skull tomography is best performed in the supine position.

52 T-tube cholangiography

a) is usually performed five days after surgery.
b) is performed with low osmolar contrast medium containing approximately 150mgs/ml iodine.
c) will demonstrate all stones present.
d) has a high incidence of minor complications.
e) may require oblique views.

53 Gadolinium

a) shortens T1 relaxivity of tissue.
b) increases signal strength in tissues on T1 weighted images.
c) decreases signal strength on T2 weighted images.
d) has eight paired electrons.
e) is not useful in mapping blood flow.

54 In radionuclide cardiac imaging

a) MUGA scans are diagnostic in all patients.
b) technetium99m labelled red blood cells are used in MUGA scans.
c) myocardial perfusion studies are a suitable alternative to exercise stress tests.
d) myocardial perfusion studies using thallium 201 require separate days for stress and exercise testing.
e) thallium 201 perfusion studies have an effective dose of more than 15 milliSieverts.

55 The following are true of angiographic technique

a) the Seldinger single wall puncture method is commonly used.
b) teflon coated guidewires have increased thrombogenicity.
c) pigtail catheters are suitable for nonselective use.
d) brachial puncture results in fewer complications.
e) pure sodium salts are the contrast agents of choice.

56 In ultrasound

a) the Fresnel zone is related to the radius of the transducer.
b) high frequency waves have superior depth resolution.
c) high frequency waves have superior depth penetration.
d) large transducers increase azimuthal resolution.
e) the intensity of the beam is uniform.

57 In the gastrointestinal tract

a) endoluminal ultrasound of the stomach is best performed with a 180° rotary transducer.
b) Tc99m DTPA is used to assess gastro-oesophageal reflux.
c) a radionuclide gastric emptying study is indicated in dumping syndrome.
d) a radionuclide bile reflux study is contraindicated in the presence of a duodenal ulcer.
e) cholecystokinin provokes bile reflux.

58 In the skull

a) the internal auditory canals are visible on a fronto-occipital 35° caudal projection.
b) the dorsum sella should not be visible on a properly positioned fronto-occipital 35° caudal projection.
c) the foramen spinosum is visible on a submentovertical view.
d) a lateral view of the mastoid bone should not be angled.
e) the median sagittal plane is at 35° for an AP view of the mastoid process.

59 In the female pelvis

a) a retroverted uterus can simulate pathological conditions.
b) the endometrial thickness should be less than 1cm premenopausally.
c) the uterus is easiest to see transabdominally when it is retroverted.
d) the normal ovarian volume varies with age.
e) the posterior cul-de-sac extends down to the posterior fornix of the vagina.

60 Within the cranium

a) arachnoid granulations are arranged around the coronal and lambdoid sutures.
b) parietal foramina transmit emissary veins of the superior sagitttal sinus.
c) the foramen rotundum contains the maxillary nerve.
d) the foramen ovale lies anterior to the foramen rotundum.
e) the clivus lies anteroinferior to the pons.

Paper Two

Answers

Paper Two   Answers

1.   a)   F
      b)   F   caudal.
      c)   T
      d)   T
      e)   F   prone; reduces eye dose.

Clark's Positioning in Radiography, Swallow et al, 11th Ed., 1986, Ch.7.

2.   a)   T
      b)   T
      c)   F   density only.
      d)   F   proportional to kVp^4.
      e)   T

Christensen's Physics of Diagnostic Radiology, Curry et al, 4th Ed., 1990, Ch.14.

3.   a)   T
      b)   T
      c)   F   perirenal space.
      d)   T
      e)   F   anterior pararenal space.

Dynamic Radiology of the Abdomen, Meyers, 4th Ed., 1993, Ch.4.

4.   a)   T
      b)   T
      c)   F
      d)   F   2·5 to 3cms.
      e)   T

An Atlas of Radiological Anatomy, Weir & Abrahams, 2nd Ed., 1986.

5.   a)   F   filtered back projection/Fourier methods.
      b)   T
      c)   F
      d)   T
      e)   T

Christensen's Physics of Diagnostic Radiology, Curry et al, 4th Ed., 1990, Ch.19.

Paper Two   Answers

6 a) T diatrizoate.
   b) F
   c) F safer in suspected aspiration.
   d) T
   e) T

Techniques in Diagnostic Imaging, Whitehouse et al, 2nd Ed., 1990, Ch.2.

7 a) F usually three.
   b) T
   c) T
   d) T
   e) F atria.

Gray's Anatomy, 38th Ed., 1995, Ch.10.

8 a) T
   b) F increases.
   c) T
   d) F unchanged.
   e) F

Radiographics, 1997, 17, 967-984.

9 a) T
   b) F increases with kV.
   c) F degrades contrast.
   d) F lower.
   e) T

Radiographics, 1996, 16, 903-916.

10 a) T
   b) T
   c) T
   d) T
   e) F no limits for patients.

Community Radiation Protection Legislation, Commission of the European Communities, 1992.

Paper Two   Answers

11 a) T
    b) T
    c) T
    d) T
    e) F

Radiographics, 1996, 16, 1165-1181.

12 a) F   posteromedial.
    b) T
    c) T
    d) F   capsule does not reach the intertrochanteric crest posteriorly.
    e) F   lateral much larger.

Gray's Anatomy, 38th Ed., 1995, Ch.6.

13 a) T
    b) T
    c) T
    d) T
    e) T

A Textbook of Radiology and Imaging, Sutton, 6th Ed., 1997, Ch.53.

14 a) F   water soluble agent if this is suspected.
    b) F   prone oblique causes variceal distension.
    c) T
    d) F
    e) F   right anterior oblique.

A Guide to Radiological Procedures, Chapman & Nakielny, 3rd Ed., 1993, Ch.3.

15 a) T   lies in floor and lateral wall.
    b) F   rarely seen clearly.
    c) F   constant in position.
    d) F   visible in 80%; inconstant.
    e) T

An Atlas of Radiological Anatomy, Weir & Abrahams, 2nd Ed., 1986.

Paper Two   Answers

16 a) T
    b) F   middle ear (tympanic cavity).
    c) T
    d) F   thin plate.
    e) F   oval window.

Gray's Anatomy, 38th Ed., 1995, Ch.8.

17 a) T
    b) F   highly vascular.
    c) F   firmly attached.
    d) T
    e) F

Gray's Anatomy, 38th Ed., 1995, Ch.8.

18 a) T
    b) F
    c) F   higher field strength better.
    d) T
    e) T

Radiographics, 1994, 14, 1083-1096.

19 a) F   none; pulsed Doppler has depth resolution.
    b) T
    c) T
    d) T   motion away gives negative shift, lower frequency.
    e) F   occurs with pulsed wave.

Radiographics, 1994, 14, 139-150.

20 a) F   two layers closely apposed but separated by venous sinuses.
    b) T
    c) T
    d) T   free border.
    e) F   all fuse and cannot be recognised individually.

Gray's Anatomy, 38th Ed., 1995, Ch.8.

Paper Two   Answers

21 a) **F**   an advantage of the procedure.
    b) **F**   requires skill.
    c) **T**
    d) **T**
    e) **F**   but reduces carbon monoxide diffusion capacity.

A Guide to Radiological Procedures, Chapman & Nakielny, 3rd Ed., 1993, Ch.10.

22 a) **F**   prone shoot-through.
    b) **T**
    c) **T**
    d) **F**   infants should be given fluids to aid visualisation.
    e) **T**   also barium studies.

Techniques in Diagnostic Imaging, Whitehouse et al, 2nd Ed., 1990, Ch.24.

23 a) **T**   but only minor.
    b) **F**   speed, contrast and base fog change; should not be used after expiry date.
    c) **F**   unhelpful due to number of components in developer.
    d) **T**
    e) **T**   ensures batch to batch stability.

Radiographics, 1997, 17, 177-187.

24 a) **T**
    b) **F**
    c) **F**
    d) **T**   if fine focus is used.
    e) **T**

Clark's Positioning in Radiography, Swallow et al, 11th Ed., 1986, Ch.1.
A Textbook of Radiology and Imaging, Sutton, 6th Ed., 1997, Ch.4.

25 a) **F**   random distribution.
    b) **F**
    c) **T**
    d) **T**
    e) **F**   must be transverse.

MRI made easy, Schild, 1990.

Paper Two   Answers

26 a) T
    b) F   highest point of tuberosity.
    c) F   caudal tilt.
    d) F   separate exposures, centring on each in turn.
    e) T   to project them off the scapula.

Clark's Positioning in Radiography, Swallow et al, 11th Ed., 1986, Ch.2.

27 a) T
    b) T
    c) F   within the pudendal canal in the lateral wall of the fossa.
    d) F   superior.
    e) F   below.

Gray's Anatomy, 38th Ed., 1995, Ch.7.

28 a) T
    b) T
    c) T
    d) T
    e) T

Gray's Anatomy, 38th Ed., 1995, Ch.13.
A Textbook of Radiology and Imaging, Sutton, 5th Ed., 1993, Ch.32.

29 a) T
    b) F   acidic compounds, inactive until ionised.
    c) T   optimally 9·8 to 10·3.
    d) T
    e) F   reduce pH.

Radiographics, 1996, 16, 1467-1479.

30 a) T
    b) T
    c) T
    d) F   occasionally absent.
    e) F   two laminae, with a central cavity which may be visualised at CT.

Gray's Anatomy, 38th Ed., 1995, Ch.8.

Paper Two   Answers

31 a) T
    b) F left.
    c) T
    d) F
    e) F internal iliac artery.

Gray's Anatomy, 38th Ed., 1995, Ch.10.

32 a) F
    b) F relates height to interspace.
    c) T
    d) T
    e) T

Christensen's Physics of Diagnostic Radiology, Curry et al, 4th Ed., 1990, Ch.8.

33 a) T
    b) T 0·4% radiographically.
    c) T
    d) F superior.
    e) F anterior.

Gray's Anatomy, 38th Ed., 1995, Ch.11.
A Textbook of Radiology and Imaging, Sutton, 5th Ed., 1993, Ch.11.

34 a) T
    b) F 3 to 5 amperes.
    c) F should be at least 2200° Celsius.
    d) T
    e) F

Christensen's Physics of Diagnostic Radiology, Curry et al, 4th Ed., 1990, Ch.2.

35 a) F vertical orientation.
    b) T
    c) T
    d) F
    e) T

Christensen's Physics of Diagnostic Radiology, Curry et al, 4th Ed., 1990, Ch.12.

Paper Two   Answers

36   a) T
     b) F   lie between gland and capsule.
     c) T
     d) F
     e) T

Gray's Anatomy, 38th Ed., 1995, Ch.15.

37   a) F
     b) T
     c) F   iodine 123 preferred.
     d) F
     e) T

Practical Nuclear Medicine, Sharp et al, 1989, Ch.16.
Making the best use of a Department of Clinical Radiology; Royal College of Radiologists London, 2nd Ed., 1993.

38   a) F   should be long enough to allow diagnostic examination.
     b) T
     c) F
     d) T
     e) F

Practical Nuclear Medicine, Sharp et al, 1989, Ch.1.

39   a) F   poor contrast.
     b) F   too viscous; toxic; may be associated with arachnoiditis.
     c) T
     d) T
     e) F

A Guide to Radiological Procedures, Chapman & Nakielny, 3rd Ed., 1993, Ch.12.

40   a) T
     b) F   high kVp, as usually a large area is being examined.
     c) T
     d) T
     e) F   finer focus should be used.

Clark's Positioning in Radiography, Swallow et al, 11th Ed., 1986, Ch.18.

Paper Two   Answers

41
a) F — two units of positive charge, the helium atom nucleus.
b) T
c) T — velocity = frequency x wavelength; velocity is constant.
d) T — sites of origin differ; x-ray outside nucleus, γ-ray inside.
e) F — but moving charged particles are deflected.

Radiographics, 1997, 17, 967-984.

42
a) T
b) T
c) T
d) F
e) T

Christensen's Physics of Diagnostic Radiology, Curry et al, 4th Ed., 1990, Ch.9.

43
a) F — superficial.
b) T
c) F — close, but not in direct contact.
d) F — left renal vein.
e) T — small veins drain body and tail.

Gray's Anatomy, 38th Ed., 1995, Ch.10.

44
a) T
b) F — lesser curve.
c) T — longitudinal, circular, oblique.
d) F — turns forwards.
e) T

Gray's Anatomy, 38th Ed., 1995, Ch.12.

45
a) T
b) T
c) F — small openings for perforating vessels and a larger one for the femoral vessels.
d) F — intracapsular.
e) T — but later becomes incorporated in it.

Gray's Anatomy, 38th Ed., 1995, Chs.6,7.

Paper Two   Answers

46
a) T
b) F   independent.
c) F   forwards at higher energies.
d) F
e) T

Christensen's Physics of Diagnostic Radiology, Curry et al, 4th Ed., 1990, Ch.4.

47
a) T
b) F   thin orbital plate.
c) T
d) F   sphenoethmoidal recess.
e) T

Gray's Anatomy, 38th Ed., 1995, Ch.11.

48
a) T
b) F   greater tuberosity.
c) T
d) F
e) T

An Atlas of Radiological Anatomy, Weir & Abrahams, 2nd Ed., 1986.

49
a) T
b) T
c) F
d) F
e) T

An Atlas of Radiological Anatomy, Weir & Abrahams, 2nd Ed., 1986.

50
a) F   posterior fornix of vagina.
b) T
c) T
d) F   medial two-thirds.
e) F   exits via inguinal ring into labium majus.

Gray's Anatomy, 38th Ed., 1995, Chs.12,14.

Paper Two   Answers

51 a) F
    b) T   also quiet breathing.
    c) T   shortest exposure time.
    d) T
    e) F   prone to diminish dose to lens.

Clark's Positioning in Radiography, Swallow et al, 11th Ed., 1986, Ch.19.

52 a) F
    b) T
    c) F
    d) F
    e) T

A Guide to Radiological Procedures, Chapman & Nakielny, 3rd Ed., 1993, Ch.4.

53 a) T
    b) T
    c) T
    d) F   seven unpaired.
    e) F

Radiographics, 1995, 15, 683-696.

54 a) F   may not be possible in arrhythmias.
    b) T
    c) T
    d) F
    e) T

Practical Nuclear Medicine, Sharp et al, 1989, Ch.9.
Making the best use of a Department of Clinical Radiology; Royal College of Radiologists London, 2nd Ed., 1993.

55 a) F
    b) T
    c) T
    d) F
    e) F

A Guide to Radiological Procedures, Chapman & Nakielny, 3rd Ed., 1993, Ch.8.

Paper Two   Answers

56 a) T   also wavelength.
    b) T
    c) F
    d) F
    e) F

Christensen's Physics of Diagnostic Radiology, Curry et al, 4th Ed., 1990, Ch.20.

57 a) F   360°.
    b) T
    c) T
    d) F
    e) T

A Guide to Radiological Procedures, Chapman & Nakielny, 3rd Ed., 1993, Ch.3.

58 a) T
    b) F   projected into foramen magnum.
    c) T
    d) F   25° caudally.
    e) T

Clark's Positioning in Radiography, Swallow et al, 11th Ed., 1986, Ch.8.

59 a) T   due to 'dropout' phenomenon at fundus.
    b) F   up to 16mms; 0·8mm postmenopausally.
    c) F   more difficult.
    d) T   also menstrual status, body habitus, pregnancy.
    e) T

Ultrasonography in Obstetrics and Gynecology, Callen, 3rd Ed., 1994, Ch.27.

60 a) F   sagittal.
    b) T
    c) T
    d) F
    e) T

Gray's Anatomy, 38th Ed., 1995, Ch.6.

Paper Three

Questions

Paper Three   Questions

1   In film processing

- a) development is an oxidation reaction.
- b) the developer has an acidic pH.
- c) thiosulphate fixer is alkaline.
- d) fog is caused by development of unexposed silver halide crystals.
- e) oxidation of the developer occurs in an infrequently used processor.

2   The following are correct of knee radiography

- a) AP views use an x-ray beam perpendicular to the film.
- b) lateral views centre to the superior border of the medial tibial condyle.
- c) horizontal beam views are usually not of diagnostic quality.
- d) the intercondylar notch is viewed in 90° and 110° flexion.
- e) inferosuperior (skyline) views of the knee are routinely used.

3   In an x-ray tube

- a) the anode is positively charged.
- b) the majority of x-rays produced are characteristic x-rays.
- c) bremsstrahlung x-rays result from the slowing down of electrons.
- d) maximum bremsstrahlung energy is determined by the tube potential.
- e) 10% of electron energy is converted to x-rays.

4   Compton scatter is

- a) the predominant reaction at low kV.
- b) responsible for less than 10% of the photons emerging from the patient.
- c) independent of atomic number.
- d) of increased significance at high kV.
- e) responsible for high energy scatter in fluoroscopy.

5   In embryology of the lungs and diaphragm

- a) the respiratory tree arises from the primitive foregut.
- b) the lung buds grow dorsally into the lateral pericardio-peritoneal canals.
- c) the diaphragm develops in part from the septum transversum.
- d) Bochdalek's hernia occurs due to failure of closure of the pleuro-peritoneal membrane.
- e) 90% of Morgagni's hernias occur in the right cardiophrenic angle.

Paper Three   Questions

6 The following are true of the diaphragm

a) both crura arise from the upper three lumbar vertebrae.
b) the aortic hiatus is the lowest and most posterior.
c) the oesophageal hiatus transmits the oesophagus and vagus nerves only.
d) there are lesser apertures in the crura.
e) the blood supply arises solely below the diaphragm.

7 In the foot

a) the head of the talus articulates with the navicular.
b) the talus has no muscle attachments.
c) the deltoid ligament attaches medially on the talus.
d) the sustentaculum tali is on the lateral border of the calcaneum.
e) the tibialis posterior tendon inserts on the navicular.

8 In paediatric urography

a) posterior urethral valves are diagnosed by retrograde urethrography.
b) if vesico-ureteric reflux is seen at micturating cystography the upper poles of the kidneys must be visualised.
c) radionuclide imaging may be used to investigate vesico-ureteric reflux.
d) a suprapubic puncture is used for cystourethrography in cases of urethral obstruction.
e) hydronephrosis is a contraindication to suprapubic puncture.

9 Regarding development of CT scanners

a) first generation scanners used a translate-rotate motion.
b) second generation scanners used a fan beam with multiple detectors.
c) third generation scanners use a rotate-rotate mechanism.
d) fourth generation scanners have a moving ring of detectors.
e) collimation is not required in spiral (helical) CT.

10 In magnetic resonance imaging

a) tissue magnetisation is easy to measure when in the direction of the external field.
b) the property of precession allows measurement of a magnetic resonance signal.
c) precession frequency is related to the nuclear magnetic field strength of an element.
d) spatial resolution does not rely on precessional frequency.
e) hydrogen spin density of cortical bone is zero.

11 At ultrasonography

a) the hepatic veins have an echogenic margin.
b) the portal vein lies posterior to the common hepatic duct.
c) it is not possible to identify the optic nerve in scans of the orbit.
d) the interhemispheric fissure is a prominent landmark in the neonatal brain.
e) the septum pellucidum is echogenic in the neonatal brain.

12 In ultrasound of the normal foetus

a) the ductus venosus enters the inferior vena cava.
b) the renal pelvis is not visible unless obstruction is present.
c) non-visualisation of the urinary bladder on a single occasion is abnormal.
d) the umbilical cord contains two veins and one artery.
e) the adrenal glands are relatively large and echo-poor.

13 In venography of the major veins

a) a bilateral cannulation technique is used.
b) the Seldinger method may be used.
c) hand injection is suboptimal.
d) injections are performed sequentially.
e) the inferior vena cava may not be visualised in small children.

14 In the large intestine

a) haustrations occur due to taeniae coli.
b) appendices epiploicae cover all of the large intestine.
c) the transverse colon has a posterior convexity.
d) the hepatic flexure is in contact with the right kidney.
e) the sigmoid colon is completely surrounded by mesentery.

15 Glucagon

a) causes gastric but not duodenal hypotonia.
b) is contraindicated in phaeochromocytoma.
c) has no effect on small bowel motility.
d) is given as a 1·5mgs intravenous dose for a barium meal.
e) causes an initial delay in gastric emptying.

Paper Three Questions

16 In the facial region

  a) a superoinferior occlusal view of the nasal bones is the best method of showing the nasal bones in children.
  b) only the side in question need be examined in mandibular injury.
  c) the symphysis menti is best shown on a PA view.
  d) dentures should be removed for a lateral view of the temporomandibular joint.
  e) zonography is adequate for tomography of the temporomandibular joint.

17 In SPECT imaging

  a) spatial resolution is superior to planar imaging.
  b) noise is reduced compared to planar imaging.
  c) perception of 3D relationships is enhanced.
  d) patient motion is less of a problem than in planar imaging.
  e) Tc99m HMPAO does not cross an intact blood-brain barrier.

18 In image quality

  a) subject contrast is increased by decreasing kV.
  b) magnification images have less noise than contact images.
  c) linear objects are more obscured by increased noise than point objects.
  d) low contrast objects are best shown on high contrast images.
  e) low contrast objects are more affected by noise than high contrast objects.

19 A gamma camera

  a) contains a scintillation crystal of pure sodium iodide.
  b) converts 90% of γ-ray energy to light.
  c) transmits light produced to photomultiplier tubes.
  d) analyses three signals to provide information.
  e) has total spatial resolution proportional to the sum of that of the collimator and the intrinsic resolution.

20 The following are true of the prostate and seminal vesicles

  a) the base of the prostate is contiguous with the base of the bladder.
  b) the anterior surface of the prostate is in direct contact with the pubic symphysis.
  c) the urethra emerges anterosuperior to the apex of the gland.
  d) the paired seminal vesicles are partly covered by peritoneum.
  e) the blood supply to the prostate is via the inferior vesical, internal pudendal and middle rectal arteries.

21 Bronchography

a) is used mainly in the investigation of bronchiectasis.
b) is performed with 25mls of low osmolar contrast medium per lung.
c) may be performed via an endotracheal tube.
d) is contraindicated in asthma.
e) has no effect on respiratory function.

22 At the wrist

a) the flexor retinaculum extends from the pisiform and hook of hamate to the scaphoid and trapezium.
b) the flexor retinaculum is crossed by the ulnar nerve and vessels.
c) all the flexor tendons run deep to the retinaculum.
d) the extensor retinaculum attaches to pisiform and triquetrum.
e) four separate synovial sheaths run beneath the extensor retinaculum.

23 In the liver and biliary system

a) the fissure for the ligamentum venosum lies posteriorly in the liver.
b) the liver is completely covered by peritoneum.
c) the inferior vena cava is closely applied to the posterior surface of the liver.
d) hepatic veins are closely related to bile ducts and hepatic artery branches.
e) the gallbladder may be separate from the liver with its own mesentery.

24 Regarding the adrenal glands

a) they lie within the renal fascia.
b) the right gland is related anteriorly to the inferior vena cava and right lobe of liver.
c) the left gland is related posteriorly to the left crus of diaphragm.
d) their blood supply is derived in part from the superior phrenic arteries.
e) accessory glands may be located in the broad ligament of the uterus.

25 With regard to radiographic film

a) the standard unit of luminance is the lumen.
b) optical density is the log of the opacity.
c) speed is the inverse of the exposure required to achieve an optical density of 2.
d) gamma is the maximum slope or gradient on the characteristic curve.
e) a higher gamma film produces more contrast.

26 In radiography of the vertebral column

a) autotomography is utilised in AP views of the cervical spine.
b) cervical ribs occur in 10% of adults.
c) the interpedicular distance is greater at L1 than L5.
d) the sagittal diameter of the lumbar spinal canal should be at least 15mms.
e) the pars interarticularis is the anterior part of the lamina.

27 Relating to the oesophagus

a) it pierces the diaphragm at the level of T10.
b) the right main bronchus causes an impression on its anterior wall.
c) it lies to the right of the aortic arch.
d) the distal oesophagus is in direct contact with the liver.
e) it has no peritoneal coverings.

28 In the shoulder

a) the rotator cuff includes the long head of triceps.
b) the long tendon of biceps passes through the shoulder capsule.
c) the fibrous capsule of the shoulder joint is lax.
d) the subacromial bursa usually connects with the shoulder joint.
e) the long head of biceps tendon has a synovial sheath.

29 The intensity of the emerging x-ray beam is

a) unaffected by filtration.
b) proportional to the milliamperage used.
c) proportional to kVp^2.
d) independent of the target material used.
e) greater with targets of low atomic number.

30 In MRI of the knee

a) the menisci have homogeneous low signal on all sequences.
b) ligaments have high signal on all sequences.
c) normal cartilage has high signal on gradient echo images.
d) bone ischaemia can be diagnosed.
e) images are usually obtained in the sagittal and axial planes.

31 Intensifying screens have

- a) a reflecting layer such as titanium dioxide in their structure.
- b) a phosphor layer of four to six centimetres thickness.
- c) a protective layer which helps prevent static electricity.
- d) phosphors which are most commonly calcium tungstate.
- e) phosphors whose main spectral emission is in the blue range.

32 Regional cerebral blood flow imaging

- a) is indicated in localisation of epileptic foci.
- b) assesses the effects of treatment regimes.
- c) can not help in distinguishing between depression and depressive dementia.
- d) is contraindicated in Huntington's disease.
- e) utilises lipophobic compounds.

33 In dental radiography

- a) the lamina dura normally appears as a dark line.
- b) intra-oral films have a lead foil backing.
- c) bite-wing films should be bent to fit the mouth curvature for a perpendicular beam.
- d) the bisecting angle technique is used for peri-apical views.
- e) an orthopantomogram gives better detail of individual teeth than intra-oral views.

34 In x-ray exposure control

- a) phototimers operate by optical density measurement.
- b) mammographic phototimers have a detector in front of the film/screen cassette.
- c) phototimers have back-up timers.
- d) automatic exposure controls typically use a single sensor.
- e) falling load generators allow short exposure times.

35 In an MRI system

- a) radiofrequency coils can only transmit or receive.
- b) gradient coils smooth out magnetic field inhomogeneities.
- c) surface coils are receivers only.
- d) shimming may be performed mechanically or electrically.
- e) the Faraday cage shields outside electrical interference.

36 Percutaneous vertebral biopsy

a) has a success rate of about 90%.
b) is safe with a platelet count of 40,000.
c) is contraindicated in suspected vascular metastases.
d) causes serious complications in 20% of cases.
e) is preferable to biopsying a lesion in the appendicular skeleton.

37 Within the brain

a) no communications occur between the cavernous sinus and the superior sagittal sinus.
b) the internal cerebral and basal veins form the great cerebral vein.
c) the thalamostriate and choroid veins form the internal cerebral vein.
d) the basal vein enters the straight sinus.
e) venous lacunae lie in the dura close to the superior sagittal sinus.

38 Shoulder arthrography

a) requires control films in the AP and lateral projections.
b) uses a landmark of 1cm above and lateral to the coracoid process for injection.
c) is indicated in adhesive capsulitis.
d) uses up to 10mls of air in double contrast studies.
e) when proceeding to CT requires further contrast injection.

39 Non-ionic water soluble contrast media

a) have an osmolarity which is 50% of that of conventional agents.
b) yield only one particle in solution.
c) are all suitable for both intravenous and intra-arterial use.
d) will only cause anaphylaxis within five minutes of administration.
e) which have a high ratio of iodine atoms to particles in solution have a better side effect profile than lower ratios.

40 Regarding the quality of magnetic resonance images

a) image detail is not affected by voxel size.
b) signal to noise ratio is highly dependent on voxel size.
c) decreasing voxel size increases spatial resolution.
d) increasing section thickness increases signal to noise ratio.
e) increasing the number of acquisitions compensates for decreased signal to noise.

41 Occipitomental views of the skull show

   a) the foramen lacerum.
   b) the foramen rotundum.
   c) the zygomaticofacial foramina.
   d) the petrous ridge.
   e) the infraorbital foramina.

42 **In the urinary tract**

   a) high density contrast medium is required for retrograde pyelography.
   b) retrograde pyelography should be halted if painful.
   c) micturating cystography is best performed in the AP projection in boys.
   d) intravasation of contrast medium is a complication of ascending urethrography.
   e) prostatic ducts are best seen at ascending (retrograde) urethrography.

43 **In the skull**

   a) parietal foramina are present in almost all patients.
   b) the optic canal contains the ophthalmic artery.
   c) the superior orbital fissure lies between the greater and lesser wings of the sphenoid.
   d) the maxillary nerve passes through the superior orbital fissure.
   e) sutural ossicles (wormian bones) do not occur in a normal skull.

44 Regarding the lymphatic system

   a) lymph nodes have several efferent vessels.
   b) peripheral lymph vessels contain valves.
   c) the cisterna chyli lies to the right of the aorta.
   d) the thoracic duct crosses right to left at the level of T2.
   e) the thoracic duct drains lymph from the right side of the thorax.

45 Regarding the trachea and bronchi

   a) the normal maximum coronal diameter of the trachea is slightly greater in women.
   b) in the neck the trachea is related to the recurrent laryngeal nerve.
   c) in the thorax, the trachea is related to the pleura on both sides.
   d) the normal carinal angle is 60 to 75 degrees.
   e) the left upper lobe bronchus has three main divisions.

46 The male urethra

a) is narrowest at the membranous segment on a urethrogram.
b) its posterior segment is usually well shown at ascending urethrography.
c) has ejaculatory ducts opening on to the verumontanum.
d) has prostatic ducts opening on to the urethral crest.
e) receives blood supply from the internal pudendal artery.

47 In the brain

a) the cerebral aqueduct connects the third and fourth ventricles.
b) the thalamus is related to the third and lateral ventricles.
c) the habenula lies posterior to the pineal gland.
d) the optic chiasm is closely related to the floor of the third ventricle.
e) the third ventricle does not contain a choroid plexus.

48 Oral cholecystography

a) iopanoic acid (Telepaque) is a suitable contrast agent.
b) is contraindicated within two weeks of intravenous cholangiography.
c) requires supine radiographs only.
d) is best performed within 14 hours of taking the contrast medium.
e) may alter thyroid function tests.

49 Tomography

a) results in an increased radiation dose to the patient.
b) utilises movement of the x-ray tube and film in opposite directions.
c) yields a slice thickness directly proportional to the amplitude of tube travel.
d) results in greater slice thickness when the angle is narrow.
e) gives increased contrast when a wide angle is used.

50 In imaging of the thyroid gland

a) ultrasound is best performed with a linear array probe of 5 to 10MHz.
b) the isthmus is poorly seen at ultrasound.
c) swallowing may enhance visualisation at ultrasound.
d) it has a high attenuation value on unenhanced CT scans.
e) it shows little enhancement on administration of contrast medium.

51 The following are true

a) hysterosalpingography is contraindicated in women who have had recurrent abortions.
b) the lacrimal duct opens into the middle meatus.
c) dacryocystography requires approximately 5mls of contrast medium.
d) the lateral meniscus of the knee is larger than the medial.
e) premature labour is a complication of amniography.

52 In the head and neck

a) the internal carotid artery is closely related to the tympanic cavity.
b) the cavernous part of the internal carotid artery lies lateral to the cranial nerves.
c) the internal carotid artery has no branches in the cavernous sinus.
d) the posterior cerebral artery arises from the basilar artery.
e) the choroidal artery is an inconstant branch of the internal carotid artery.

53 Characteristics of ultrasound waves include

a) the ability to travel in a vacuum.
b) movement in longitudinal waves.
c) frequency in the range 1 to 20MHz.
d) velocity in soft tissue of 1540 metres/second.
e) velocity in soft tissue which is independent of tissue density.

54 In radiography of the heart

a) the cardiothoracic ratio relates the maximum transverse diameter of the heart to the transverse width of the thorax at the costophrenic angles.
b) a cardiothoracic ratio of greater than 50% is abnormal in a child.
c) the left anterior oblique position optimises visualisation of the aortic arch.
d) mitral valve calcification is best assessed on a PA film.
e) barium studies are helpful in cardiac assessment.

55 A barium enema

a) should always demonstrate the whole colon.
b) is contraindicated following recent rectal biopsy.
c) is safe in toxic megacolon if performed slowly.
d) has a mortality of 80% if venous intravasation occurs.
e) requires the usual preparation in patients with acute ulcerative colitis.

56 Regarding the basal ganglia

a) the caudate nucleus is completely separate from the lentiform.
b) the globus pallidus lies medially in the lentiform nucleus.
c) the lateral striate artery runs on the lateral aspect of the lentiform nucleus.
d) the insula lies laterally.
e) the internal capsule is convex laterally.

57 In the venous system

a) bronchial veins enter the main pulmonary vein.
b) an inferior vena cavogram requires bilateral injections.
c) the Valsalva manoeuvre causes retrograde filling of tributaries at inferior vena cavography.
d) the calf vein anatomy is relatively constant.
e) portal vein tributaries do not contain valves in adults.

58 In x-ray tube technology

a) tungsten is a good conductor of heat.
b) rotating anodes have a greater x-ray output than fixed anodes.
c) focal spot size increases with increasing anode angle.
d) beam intensity is lower on the cathode side of the beam.
e) the heel effect is utilised in mammography.

59 In the pelvis

a) weight bearing views improve the assessment of symphysis subluxation.
b) the central ray is tilted caudally in supine AP views of the sacroiliac joints.
c) supine AP views of the sacroiliac joints require more tilt of the central beam in men.
d) a PA view of both sacroiliac joints does not require tube tilt.
e) posterior oblique views of a sacroiliac joint examine the side raised from the table.

60 In the photographic process

a) smaller halide grains have higher photographic speed.
b) latent image in exposed grains catalyses development.
c) development of unexposed halide grains contributes to fog.
d) higher development temperature decreases the amount of fog.
e) latent image fade occurs if there is a long delay between exposure and development.

Paper Three

Answers

Paper Three Answers

1 a) F reduction.
   b) F alkaline.
   c) F acidic.
   d) T
   e) T

Christensen's Physics of Diagnostic Radiology, Curry et al, 4th Ed., 1990, Ch.10.

2 a) F perpendicular to tibia; slight tilt to film.
   b) T
   c) F
   d) F beam at 90° and 110° to the tibial axis.
   e) F flexion may exacerbate injury.

Clark's Positioning in Radiography, Swallow et al, 11th Ed., 1986, Ch.3.

3 a) T cathode negative.
   b) F bremsstrahlung mostly.
   c) T 'braking' radiation.
   d) T incident electrons colliding with nucleus give up all their energy.
   e) F 1%; 99% heat.

Radiographics, 1997, 17, 967-984.

4 a) F photoelectric effect.
   b) F 50 to 90%.
   c) T
   d) T
   e) T

Christensen's Physics of Diagnostic Radiology, Curry et al, 4th Ed., 1990, Ch.5.

5 a) T
   b) T
   c) T
   d) T
   e) T due to developmental defect between septum transversum and costal origins of diaphragm.

Gray's Anatomy, 38th Ed., 1995, Ch.3.
A Textbook of Radiology and Imaging, Sutton, 5th Ed., 1993, Ch.12.

Paper Three Answers

6
- a) **F** left from upper two only.
- b) **T**
- c) **F** also branches of left gastric artery and gastric nerves.
- d) **T** for splanchnic nerves.
- e) **F** also branches of internal thoracic artery.

Gray's Anatomy, 38th Ed., 1995, Ch.7.

7
- a) **T**
- b) **T**
- c) **T**
- d) **F** medial.
- e) **T**

Gray's Anatomy, 38th Ed., 1995, Ch.6.

8
- a) **F** requires antegrade study.
- b) **T**
- c) **T**
- d) **T**
- e) **F**

Techniques in Diagnostic Imaging, Whitehouse et al, 2nd Ed., 1990, Ch.24.

9
- a) **T**
- b) **T**
- c) **T**
- d) **F** fixed.
- e) **F** related to area of interest.

Christensen's Physics of Diagnostic Radiology, Curry et al, 4th Ed., 1990, Ch.19.
Radiographics, 1994, 14, 887-893.

10
- a) **F** because it is so small.
- b) **T**
- c) **T** precession frequency = gyromagnetic ratio of nucleus x external magnetic field strength.
- d) **F** differences in precessional frequency allow spatial resolution.
- e) **T** highest for fluids.

Radiographics, 1994, 14, 829-846.

Paper Three   Answers

11 a) F   portal veins.
    b) T
    c) F
    d) T
    e) T

An Atlas of Radiological Anatomy, Weir & Abrahams, 2nd Ed., 1986.

12 a) T
    b) F
    c) F
    d) F   two arteries, one vein.
    e) T

Ultrasonography in Obstetrics and Gynecology, Callen, 3rd Ed., 1994, Chs.16,18,20.

13 a) T
    b) T
    c) F   but should be rapid.
    d) F
    e) T

A Guide to Radiological Procedures, Chapman & Nakielny, 3rd Ed., 1993, Ch.9.

14 a) T
    b) F   do not cover caecum, appendix, rectum.
    c) F   anterior convexity.
    d) T
    e) T   the sigmoid mesocolon.

Gray's Anatomy, 38th Ed., 1995, Ch.12.

15 a) F
    b) T
    c) T
    d) F   0·15mg.
    e) T

Techniques in Diagnostic Imaging, Whitehouse et al, 2nd Ed., 1990, Ch.3.
Pharmaco-radiology in barium examinations with special reference to glucagon, British Journal of Radiology, 1975, 48, 691-703.

Paper Three   Answers

16 a) F   often cannot demonstrate the nasal bone adequately.
    b) F   both sides to exclude contre-coup fracture.
    c) F   best on anterior oblique.
    d) F
    e) T

Clark's Positioning in Radiography, Swallow et al, 11th Ed., 1986, Ch.10.

17 a) F
    b) F
    c) T
    d) F   motion artefacts simulate perfusion defects.
    e) F   freely diffuses across on first pass.

Radiographics, 1996, 16, 661-668.

18 a) T
    b) T
    c) F   point objects, because there is less to be obscured.
    d) T
    e) T

Radiographics, 1997, 17, 479-498.

19 a) F   contains traces of thallium.
    b) F   approximately 10%.
    c) T
    d) T
    e) F   sum of the squares.

Practical Nuclear Medicine, Sharp et al, 1989, Chs.2,3.

20 a) T
    b) F   separated by a venous plexus.
    c) T
    d) T
    e) T

Gray's Anatomy, 38th Ed., 1995, Ch.14.

Paper Three   Answers

---

21 a) T
b) F   25mls total maximum volume.
c) T
d) F
e) F

A Guide to Radiological Procedures, Chapman & Nakielny, 3rd Ed., 1993, Ch.7.

22 a) T
b) T
c) F   palmaris longus and flexor carpi ulnaris lie superficially.
d) T
e) F   six.

Gray's Anatomy, 38th Ed., 1995, Ch.7.

23 a) T
b) F
c) T   may lie in a tunnel of liver.
d) F   portal veins are.
e) T

Gray's Anatomy, 38th Ed., 1995, Ch.12.

24 a) T
b) T
c) T
d) F   inferior phrenic.
e) T

Gray's Anatomy, 38th Ed., 1995, Ch.15.

25 a) F   nit.
b) T
c) F   optical density of 1 above base plus fog.
d) T
e) T

Radiographics, 1996, 16, 903-916.

Paper Three   Answers

26
- a) T — to blur out the mandibular shadow.
- b) F — 0·5 to 1%.
- c) F — normally increases from L1 to L5.
- d) T
- e) T

An Atlas of Radiological Anatomy, Weir & Abrahams, 2nd Ed., 1986.

27
- a) T
- b) F — left main bronchus.
- c) T
- d) T — grooves the posterior aspect of the left lobe.
- e) F — distal part is covered anteriorly and on the left side.

Gray's Anatomy, 38th Ed., 1995, Ch.12.

28
- a) F — supraspinatus, infraspinatus, teres minor, subscapularis.
- b) T
- c) T — to allow movement.
- d) F
- e) T

Gray's Anatomy, 38th Ed., 1995, Ch.6.

29
- a) F
- b) T
- c) T
- d) F
- e) F

Christensen's Physics of Diagnostic Radiology, Curry et al, 4th Ed., 1990, Ch.2.

30
- a) T
- b) F
- c) T
- d) T
- e) F — sagittal and coronal.

A Textbook of Radiology and Imaging, Sutton, 5th Ed., 1993, Ch.4.

Paper Three Answers

31 a) T also magnesium oxide.
    b) F four to six millimetres.
    c) T
    d) T
    e) T

Christensen's Physics of Diagnostic Radiology, Curry et al, 4th Ed., 1990, Ch.9.

32 a) T
    b) T
    c) F may be of help but is not specific.
    d) F
    e) F lipophilic, e.g. HMPAO (hexamethylpropyleneamineoxime)

A Guide to Radiological Procedures, Chapman & Nakielny, 3rd Ed., 1993, Ch.12.

33 a) F dense white line.
    b) T tube side must be carefully checked.
    c) F causes pressure marks on films.
    d) T
    e) F not as well defined.

Clark's Positioning in Radiography, Swallow et al, 11th Ed., 1986, Ch.11.

34 a) T
    b) F behind - to avoid artefact on film.
    c) T in case of failure of detector or circuit.
    d) F usually three.
    e) T

Radiographics, 1997, 17, 1533-1557.

35 a) F can do both.
    b) F
    c) T
    d) T
    e) F radio waves.

MRI made easy, Schild, 1990.

Paper Three   Answers

36
a) T
b) F
c) F   may be performed but a fine needle should be used.
d) F   rare, 0·2%.
e) F

A Guide to Radiological Procedures, Chapman & Nakielny, 3rd Ed., 1993, Ch.12.

37
a) F   via superior anastomotic and middle cerebral veins.
b) F   two internal cerebral veins form the great cerebral vein (of Galen).
c) T
d) F   enters great cerebral vein.
e) T

Gray's Anatomy, 38th Ed., 1995, Ch.10.

38
a) F
b) F   1cm below and lateral.
c) T
d) T
e) F

A Guide to Radiological Procedures, Chapman & Nakielny, 3rd Ed., 1993, Ch.11.

39
a) T
b) T
c) F
d) F   can occur up to 30 minutes after use.
e) T

Techniques in Diagnostic Imaging, Whitehouse et al, 2nd Ed., 1990, Ch.30.

40
a) F   image detail highly dependent on voxel size.
b) T
c) T   but at the expense of signal to noise.
d) T   but with loss of detail in image.
e) T

Radiographics, 1995, 15, 683-696.

Paper Three   Answers

41 a) F
    b) T
    c) T
    d) F
    e) T

An Atlas of Radiological Anatomy, Weir & Abrahams, 2nd Ed., 1986.

42 a) F   if too dense, it obscures small lesions.
    b) T   may be possible to adjust catheter position.
    c) F   oblique better.
    d) T
    e) F   descending (micturating) urethrography.

A Guide to Radiological Procedures, Chapman & Nakielny, 3rd Ed., 1993, Ch.5.

43 a) F   40 to 60% depending on race.
    b) T
    c) T
    d) F   inferior orbital fissure.
    e) F

Gray's Anatomy, 38th Ed., 1995, Ch.6.

44 a) F   single efferent, several afferents.
    b) T
    c) T
    d) F   T5.
    e) T

Gray's Anatomy, 38th Ed., 1995, Ch.10.
A Textbook of Radiology and Imaging, Sutton, 5th Ed., 1993, Ch.27.

45 a) F   21mms in women; 25mms in men.
    b) T
    c) F   only on the right.
    d) T
    e) F   two; anterior, apicoposterior.

Gray's Anatomy, 38th Ed., 1995, Ch.11.
A Textbook of Radiology and Imaging, Sutton, 6th Ed., 1997, Ch.11.

Paper Three   Answers

46
a) T
b) F
c) T
d) F   open into the prostatic sinus lateral to the crest.
e) T   via urethral artery.

Gray's Anatomy, 38th Ed., 1995, Chs.10,13.
A Textbook of Radiology and Imaging, Sutton, 5th Ed., 1993, Ch.42.

47
a) T
b) T
c) F
d) T
e) F   has one in each side of its roof.

Gray's Anatomy, 38th Ed., 1995, Ch.8.

48
a) T
b) F   one week.
c) F
d) T
e) T

A Guide to Radiological Procedures, Chapman & Nakielny, 3rd Ed., 1993, Ch.4.

49
a) T
b) T
c) F   inverse relationship.
d) T   zonography.
e) F

Christensen's Physics of Diagnostic Radiology, Curry et al, 4th Ed., 1990, Ch.16.

50
a) T
b) F
c) T   especially for retrosternal extension.
d) T
e) F

A Textbook of Radiology and Imaging, Sutton, 6th Ed., 1997, Ch.46.
A Guide to Radiological Procedures, Chapman & Nakielny, 3rd Ed., 1993, Ch.15.

51	a)	F	
	b)	F	inferior meatus.
	c)	F	2mls usually enough.
	d)	F	
	e)	T	

An Atlas of Radiological Anatomy, Weir & Abrahams, 2nd Ed., 1986.

52	a)	T	
	b)	F	
	c)	F	numerous small branches.
	d)	T	
	e)	F	small, but constant.

Gray's Anatomy, 38th Ed., 1995, Ch.10.

53	a)	F
	b)	T
	c)	T
	d)	T
	e)	F

Christensen's Physics of Diagnostic Radiology, Curry et al, 4th Ed., 1990, Ch.20.

54	a)	F	usually above costophrenic angles.
	b)	F	up to 60% is considered normal.
	c)	T	
	d)	F	lateral film or fluoroscopy.
	e)	T	

Clark's Positioning in Radiography, Swallow et al, 11th Ed., 1986, Ch.13.
A Textbook of Radiology and Imaging, Sutton, 6th Ed., 1997, Ch.20.

55	a)	F	not with tight stricture.
	b)	T	although some proceed after biopsy through flexible scope.
	c)	F	toxic megacolon is an absolute contraindication.
	d)	T	
	e)	F	instant enema may suffice due to empty colon in active disease.

A Guide to Radiological Procedures, Chapman & Nakielny, 3rd Ed., 1993, Ch.3.

Paper Three   Answers

56 a) F   fuses inferiorly with the putamen.
    b) T   putamen laterally.
    c) T   and pierces its substance.
    d) T
    e) F   concave.

Gray's Anatomy, 38th Ed., 1995, Ch.8.

57 a) T   deep bronchial veins; superficial drain to the azygos and hemiazygos veins.
    b) T   both femoral veins.
    c) T
    d) F   wide variation.
    e) T

An Atlas of Radiological Anatomy, Weir & Abrahams, 2nd Ed., 1986.

58 a) F
    b) T   due to higher heat loading available.
    c) T   due to geometry.
    d) F   anode side.
    e) T   cathode side of tube aligned to chest wall of patient.

Radiographics, 1997, 17, 1259-1268.

59 a) T
    b) F
    c) F   females.
    d) F   caudal tilt.
    e) T

Clark's Positioning in Radiography, Swallow et al, 11th Ed., 1986, Ch.4.

60 a) F   larger grains are faster.
    b) T
    c) T
    d) F   increases.
    e) T

Radiographics, 1996, 16, 1467-1479.

Paper Four

Questions

1 Regarding the parathyroid glands

a) normal glands cannot be identified at CT.
b) false positive results do not occur in technetium/thallium scanning.
c) they enhance on administration of intravenous contrast medium.
d) parathormone assays require sampling of multiple veins.
e) radiation dose to the thyroid is negligible during CT.

2 With regard to the kidneys

a) their long axis is inferolateral and the transverse axis posteromedial.
b) the right kidney lies approximately 1·25cms lower than the left.
c) the renal hila lie at the level of the transpyloric plane.
d) the most anterior structure at the hilum is the renal artery.
e) the left renal vein courses posterior to the splenic vein and anterior to the aorta.

3 Regarding filtration of the x-ray beam

a) inherent tube filtration is more than 1·5mms aluminium equivalent.
b) most inherent filtration occurs at the envelope of the glass tube.
c) added filtration is required to be at least 2·5mms aluminium equivalent at 70kVp or more.
d) aluminium filtration decreases the mean energy of the beam.
e) heavy metal filters increase contrast.

4 Rare earth screens

a) have an intrinsic conversion efficiency of 20%.
b) have a higher absorption capacity than calcium tungstate screens.
c) absorb photons by the photoelectric effect.
d) consist of pure crystals of the phosphors.
e) have K edges which are higher than that of tungsten.

5 The following are true of barium preparations

a) their use is contraindicated in cases of suspected pleural or peritoneal perforation.
b) a concentration of 100% weight/volume is suitable for barium swallows.
c) a medium density high viscosity preparation is used for barium meals.
d) flocculation is increased in the presence of mucin.
e) dimethylpolysiloxane is an anti-flocculant.

6 In the imaging of back pain and sciatica

a) disc prolapse occurs at L4/5 or L5/S1 levels in 90% of cases.
b) degenerative disease on plain films correlates well with symptomatology.
c) facet joints are richly innervated.
d) myelography is the best modality for assessment of lateral disc prolapse.
e) imaging can not distinguish recurrent disc prolapse from epidural fibrosis.

7 In magnetic resonance imaging

a) tissue magnetisation is proportional to hydrogen spin density.
b) contrast is not related to tissue relaxation parameters.
c) T1 describes spin-lattice relaxation.
d) tissue T2 is much longer than T1.
e) tissue T1 and T2 increase with increased water content.

8 Regarding the thyroid gland

a) it lies at the level of C5 to T1.
b) the isthmus lies anterior to the second and third tracheal rings.
c) the pyramidal lobe, when present, usually arises from the right lobe.
d) the external laryngeal nerve lies on its medial aspect.
e) the thyroidea ima artery arises from the internal carotid artery.

9 In the nose

a) the bony framework is solely from the nasal bones.
b) the nasal septum is purely cartilaginous.
c) the nasal conchae have corresponding inferolateral meati.
d) the nasolacrimal duct opens into the inferior meatus.
e) the frontal sinus is the most anterior opening in the middle meatus.

10 In quality control

a) a control chart plots values of interest against time.
b) a control chart does not allow evaluation of trends.
c) in film processing the specified operating level should not be adjusted if quality control values are consistently above or below it.
d) the base-plus-fog level requires upper and lower control limits.
e) film used for testing should be the same as for clinical work.

11 In intervention in the gastrointestinal tract

a) a tracheo-oesophageal fistula contraindicates balloon dilatation of the oesophagus.
b) low osmolar contrast medium should be used for assessment of stricture prior to oesophageal dilatation.
c) air reduction of intussusception is slower than with barium.
d) in children over four years reduction of intussusception is best performed with air.
e) treatment of meconium ileus with water soluble contrast medium is contraindicated in the presence of a volvulus.

12 In the abdomen

a) the ligamentum teres separates the left and right lobes of the liver.
b) the caudate lobe of the liver is adjacent to the inferior vena cava.
c) the spleen is extraperitoneal.
d) accessory spleens are found in 10 to 30% of autopsies.
e) the uncinate process of the pancreas lies in front of the mesenteric vessels.

13 Regarding muscles around the hip joint

a) quadratus femoris is in direct contact with the joint posteriorly.
b) piriformis is in direct contact with the joint capsule.
c) rectus femoris arises from the capsule.
d) obturator internus lies inferior to the joint.
e) pectineus separates the joint capsule from the femoral vessels.

14 CT scanners

a) operate at a constant kV.
b) can have tube currents of 600mA or more.
c) have a single collimation device.
d) now use a scintillation detector which is typically sodium iodide.
e) of any generation may use either a scintillation or xenon detector.

15 In cervical spine radiography

a) routine views deliver an effective dose of 0·1 milliSievert.
b) lateral views of C1 to C7 centre to C4.
c) AP views of C1 to C7 use caudally angled beams.
d) posterior oblique views demonstrate the foramina nearer the film.
e) flexion and extension views are performed with a horizontal beam.

Paper Four   Questions

16 Regarding radiation workers

- a) the dose limit for whole body exposure is 50 milliSieverts (5 rems) per annum.
- b) women of reproductive capacity should not receive more than 13 milliSieverts (1·3 rems) in a quarter.
- c) once pregnancy is declared, the accumulated dose to the foetus must not exceed 10 milliSieverts (1 rem).
- d) planned special exposures can be safely performed by category A and B workers.
- e) the dose rate from a cathode ray tube should not be more than 5 microSieverts per hour at 0·05 metres.

17 In the central nervous system

- a) cervical myelography is useful in the investigation of raised intracranial pressure.
- b) the foramen of Magendie is in the midline of the fourth ventricle.
- c) the interpeduncular cistern lies behind the dorsum sella.
- d) the third ventricle does not contain a choroid plexus.
- e) the pineal recess lies in the posterior aspect of the third ventricle.

18 In the cerebrum

- a) the corpus callosum connects the cerebral hemispheres.
- b) olfactory nerves perforate the cribriform plate.
- c) the hippocampus lies in the floor of the body of the lateral ventricle.
- d) Broca's area lies in the anterior aspect of the occipital cortex.
- e) the temporal lobe is concerned with hearing.

19 With regard to the abdominal muscles

- a) quadratus lumborum is crossed by the gonadal veins.
- b) psoas major contributes to the medial arcuate ligament of the diaphragm.
- c) psoas minor is entirely intra-abdominal.
- d) the muscles of the anterior abdominal wall all contribute to the linea alba.
- e) rectus abdominis has a single tendinous origin.

20 In the photographic process

- a) silver halide is most sensitive to light at the red end of the spectrum.
- b) spectral dyes allow use of green light.
- c) panchromatic film is sensitive to light over the entire visible spectrum.
- d) cubic silver halide grains are used in mammography film.
- e) gold and sulphur are used to sensitise grains.

21 In an x-ray spectrum

a) quality refers to the energy distribution of the beam.
b) a high quality beam gives a higher dose to the patient than lower quality.
c) the quantity of x-rays present is proportional to the tube potential squared.
d) characteristic radiation for tungsten occurs at 60keV.
e) a change in exposure time alters the shape.

22 In radionuclide bone imaging

a) technetium99m labelled phosphate analogues are frequently used.
b) the radionuclide is excreted by the kidneys.
c) 50 to 60% of the nuclide accumulates in bone.
d) an effective dose of 1 milliSievert or less is delivered.
e) a three phase scan obtains images at two, four and 24 hours post injection.

23 Regarding the ovaries

a) the mesovarium attaches to the anterior aspect of the broad ligament.
b) they occupy the ovarian fossa which is bound by the ureter and internal iliac artery in the nulliparous state.
c) the ovarian ligament runs from the inferior ovarian surface to the uterus.
d) the ovarian vessels run in the suspensory ligament of the ovary.
e) the ovarian artery lies anterior to the fallopian tube.

24 In the arterial system

a) the left subclavian artery lies against the lung.
b) an aberrant right subclavian artery passes anterior to the trachea and oesophagus.
c) the right renal artery passes in front of the inferior vena cava.
d) the hepatic artery crosses anterior to the portal vein.
e) the gastroduodenal artery lies anterior to the neck of the pancreas.

25 In a normal pregnancy

a) the foetal spine has three ossification centres.
b) cartilaginous parts of bone are not identifiable sonographically.
c) head circumference is an appropriate parameter for evaluating growth.
d) thoracic circumference is not useful in assessing growth.
e) placental thickness correlates loosely with menstrual age.

Paper Four Questions

26 Gadolinium

a) is paramagnetic.
b) is toxic in its free state.
c) is administered intravenously only.
d) shortens tissue T1 and T2.
e) is best used for T2 weighted images.

27 In lymphangiography

a) lymphatic vessels contain valves.
b) a lower limb examination should be terminated when contrast medium reaches the thoracic duct.
c) crossover of lymphatic vessels occurs normally in the pelvis.
d) the cisterna chyli lies at the T11-T12 level.
e) contrast medium can stay in lymph nodes for up to eighteen months.

28 In radiography of the shoulder region

a) for a lateral view of the humeral head a line joining the humeral epicondyles should be parallel to the film.
b) an AP view of the shoulder is centred to the palpable coracoid process.
c) an inferosuperior view is centred to the coracoid process.
d) an inferosuperior view is best performed in the erect position.
e) a gleno-humeral AP view requires rotation of the patient to the affected side.

29 Within the heart

a) the venae cavae enter the anterior aspect of the right atrium.
b) the coronary sinus enters the left atrium.
c) an axial section of the right ventricle is crescentic in shape.
d) the orifice of the left atrioventricular valve is much larger than the right.
e) the left atrium is larger than the right.

30 The following are true of the photographic properties of x-ray film

a) film density is the ratio of incident to transmitted light.
b) the characteristic curve relates optical density to the log of the relative exposure.
c) at zero exposure film density is zero.
d) speed is directly related to exposure.
e) film latitude is the range of log relative exposures yielding an acceptable density within the diagnostic range.

31 The following are true of the lungs

a) bronchial vessels are the most posterior structures at the hilum.
b) the right pulmonary artery is anteroinferior to the right main bronchus.
c) the thoracic duct crosses anterior to the left main bronchus.
d) the lingular bronchus arises from the left lower lobe bronchus.
e) the bronchial arteries arise from the aorta and intercostal vessels.

32 In the venous system

a) the cephalic vein lies on the lateral aspect of the arm.
b) the thoracic duct enters the left subclavian vein at its junction with the internal jugular vein.
c) the azygos vein ascends along the left border of the spine.
d) the pulmonary veins lie above the pulmonary arteries.
e) the internal vertebral venous plexuses are extradural.

33 In the abdomen

a) the epiploic foramen connects the greater and lesser peritoneal sacs.
b) the urinary bladder is mostly intraperitoneal.
c) the lesser sac (omental bursa) lies behind the stomach.
d) the root of the mesentery runs behind the horizontal part of the duodenum.
e) the root of the mesentery crosses the aorta.

34 In x-ray tube technology

a) efficiency of x-ray production increases as kV is increased.
b) increase in mA changes the quality of the x-ray beam.
c) filtration alters the shape of the x-ray spectrum.
d) heel effect is least in the direction of the anode-cathode axis.
e) heel effect causes approximately 5% variation in intensity.

35 In the forearm and hand

a) the ulnar styloid normally projects beyond the radial styloid.
b) the pisiform articulates with the triquetral only.
c) the trapezoid lies in the proximal row of carpal bones.
d) the hamate hook forms part of the medial wall of the carpal tunnel.
e) ossification occurs earlier in females.

36 In the skull base

a) the accessory meningeal artery passes through the foramen ovale.
b) the middle meningeal artery passes through the foramen ovale.
c) the foramina ovale and spinosum are occasionally confluent.
d) the internal carotid artery passes through the foramen lacerum.
e) the hypoglossal canal carries an artery, vein and nerve.

37 Radionuclide lung scanning

a) is contraindicated in the presence of a left to right shunt.
b) uses macro-aggregated albumen (MAA) particles from 10 to 100 micrometres in size.
c) using technetium99m DTPA allows simultaneous ventilation and perfusion imaging.
d) a pinhole collimator is generally used.
e) delivers an effective dose of 1·2 milliSieverts in perfusion studies.

38 In the gastrointestinal tract

a) Buscopan causes gastric dilatation.
b) Buscopan acts for approximately three hours after intravenous injection.
c) typical intravenous dose of glucagon for a barium enema in an adult is 1·0mg.
d) glucagon increases small bowel transit time.
e) metoclopramide has extrapyramidal side effects.

39 In paediatric radiology

a) gridless screening is advised to decrease radiation dose.
b) radiographic detail is lost when a grid is not used.
c) sedation is used routinely.
d) room humidity and temperature need not be tightly controlled as most tests are of short duration.
e) neonates are more susceptible to radiation damage than the foetus.

40 Ultrasound transducers

a) usually contain two piezoelectric crystals.
b) have a resonant frequency dependent on the crystal thickness.
c) have a backing block which absorbs returning sound waves.
d) have a Q factor which is constant.
e) can send and receive simultaneously.

41 Regarding the vascular supply of the brain

a) the posterior communicating artery connects the anterior and posterior cerebral arteries.
b) the corpus striatum and internal capsule are supplied by the middle cerebral artery.
c) the choroid plexuses of the third and lateral ventricles are supplied by the internal carotid and posterior cerebral arteries.
d) the intracerebral veins contain valves.
e) the brachial vein drains into the petrosal vein.

42 In embryology of the gastrointestinal tract

a) the lesser omentum arises from the ventral mesogastrium.
b) the pancreas arises entirely from the dorsal pancreatic bud.
c) the dorsal mesogastrium forms the posterior wall of the lesser sac.
d) the spleen forms in the ventral mesogastrium.
e) the liver is derived from the endoderm of the foregut.

43 Intravenous cholangiography

a) is suitably performed using meglumine ioglycamate (Biligram).
b) will clearly visualise the biliary tract when serum bilirubin levels are greater than 60 micromoles/litre.
c) utilises a bolus injection technique in preference to infusion methods.
d) iotroxate is superior to ioglycamate for infusion.
e) causes altered liver function which is not dose related.

44 In the production of x-rays

a) kinetic energy is converted into electromagnetic radiation.
b) characteristic x-rays occur over a continuous spectrum.
c) the quantity produced is proportional to the square root of the tube potential.
d) voltage waveform does not affect x-ray quantity.
e) the x-ray spectrum is affected by the atomic number of the anode.

45 The heel effect

a) is more pronounced on the cathode side of the x-ray tube.
b) is more pronounced at increased focus-film distances.
c) is less pronounced on smaller films at fixed focus-film distances.
d) causes a non-uniform beam.
e) has no practical applications.

46 A PA20 view of the skull shows the following well

a) the foramen rotundum.
b) the infra-orbital foramina.
c) the frontal sinuses.
d) the ethmoid sinuses.
e) the internal auditory canals.

47 Tomography of the larynx

a) is best performed in the lateral projection.
b) shows adducted true cords when phonating 'EE'.
c) demonstrates the laryngeal ventricle.
d) will not help in diagnosing cord paralysis.
e) shows the true cords to be at a higher level than the false cords.

48 The following are true of subject contrast

a) it is affected by both subject thickness and density.
b) it is independent of atomic number.
c) it is primarily due to the photoelectric effect.
d) low kVp techniques maximise contrast.
e) it can be expressed as the log of the ratio of beam intensity through thick and thin parts.

49 Collimators in nuclear medicine

a) consist of lead plates with septa.
b) provide a means of determining site of origin of the γ-ray.
c) minify the image, when converging in type.
d) have a sensitivity which is decreased by an increased number of septa.
e) have resolution which is increased by thicker septa.

50 Metoclopramide

a) is used as a hurrying agent.
b) decreases gastric emptying.
c) has no effect on the appearance of small bowel.
d) is used intravenously and orally.
e) when used orally is given at the same time as the barium.

51 Portal venography

a) may be performed directly or indirectly.
b) is usually a day case procedure.
c) is performed by hand injection of approximately 50mls of contrast medium into the spleen.
d) will always opacify a patent portal vein.
e) is contraindicated if there is a large amount of ascites.

52 Hysterosalpingography

a) is indicated in the investigation of infertility.
b) causes tubal spasm which is relieved by octyl nitrite.
c) is best performed with oily contrast medium.
d) can cause abortion.
e) requires approximately 50mls of contrast medium.

53 The photoelectric effect

a) involves complete absorption of the incident photon.
b) is directly proportional to the energy of the incident photon.
c) is proportional to Z^3.
d) enhances natural tissue contrast.
e) contributes little to patient dose.

54 In the thorax

a) normal diaphragmatic movement is approximately 2·5 to 5cms.
b) posterior oblique views of ribs should be performed with a perpendicular beam.
c) cervical ribs may require a caudally angled coned AP view.
d) an anterior oblique view of the sternum requires suspended respiration.
e) a long exposure time is used for an anterior oblique view of the sternum.

55 In MRI of the shoulder

a) surface coils are used.
b) normal tendons have low signal.
c) fluid in bursae has low signal on T2 weighted images.
d) calcification is easily evaluated.
e) STIR or T2 weighting are useful.

56 The following are true of the muscles of mastication

a) they are supplied by the mandibular nerve.
b) the parotid duct crosses deep to masseter.
c) temporalis lies superficial to the maxillary artery.
d) lateral pterygoid has a single site of origin.
e) medial pterygoid is related medially to the styloid muscles.

57 Regarding screen-film performance

a) the reciprocity law does not apply to screen-produced light.
b) screen-film speed is not affected by film processing.
c) high modulation transfer function indicates less blurring.
d) noise has no effect on image sharpness.
e) mammography film has higher spatial resolution than other diagnostic film.

58 For the quality of images in magnetic resonance

a) decreasing section thickness improves image detail.
b) decreasing TR increases T1 weighting.
c) tissue T1 is independent of magnetic field strength.
d) heavily T2 weighted spin echo is the most sensitive method of detecting lesions without contrast agents.
e) increasing TE increases T2 weighting.

59 In x-ray tubes

a) beryllium is used for the window in mammography tubes.
b) the anode stem transmits considerable heat to the rotor bearings.
c) leaked radiation is all contained within the tube housing.
d) the focal spot is larger at higher filament currents.
e) mammography tubes typically operate at 25 to 30kVp.

60 In radiography of foreign bodies

a) foreign bodies in the soft tissues are best shown with a low kV technique.
b) ingested non-opaque foreign bodies can be demonstrated by barium studies.
c) a single PA chest film is adequate for assessment of complications of inhaled foreign bodies.
d) all ocular foreign bodies are of high attenuation at CT.
e) the limbal ring method is a simple non-invasive technique for localising an ocular foreign body.

Paper Four

Answers

Paper Four   Answers

1. a) T
   b) F
   c) T
   d) T
   e) F

A Textbook of Radiology and Imaging, Sutton, 5th Ed., 1993, Ch. 46.

2. a) T
   b) T
   c) T
   d) F   renal vein.
   e) T

Gray's Anatomy, 38th Ed., 1995, Chs. 10, 13.

3. a) F   0·5-1mm.
   b) T
   c) T
   d) F
   e) T

Christensen's Physics of Diagnostic Radiology, Curry et al, 4th Ed., 1990, Ch. 6.

4. a) T
   b) T
   c) T
   d) F   they require activators.
   e) F

Christensen's Physics of Diagnostic Radiology, Curry et al, 4th Ed., 1990, Ch. 9.

5. a) T
   b) T
   c) F   low viscosity agents.
   d) T
   e) F   anti-foaming agent.

Techniques in Diagnostic Imaging, Whitehouse et al, 2nd Ed., 1990, Chs. 2 to 5.

Paper Four   Answers

6 a) T   90 to 95%.
   b) F
   c) T
   d) F   CT or MRI needed.
   e) F   contrast enhanced CT or MRI can.

A Guide to Radiological Procedures, Chapman & Nakielny, 3rd Ed., 1993, Ch.12.

7 a) T   the amount of detectable hydrogen in each voxel.
   b) F   T1 and T2 are the main determinants of image contrast.
   c) T
   d) F   shorter.
   e) T

Radiographics, 1994, 14, 829-846.

8 a) T
   b) T
   c) F   from the isthmus or left lobe.
   d) T
   e) F   aortic arch or brachiocephalic trunk.

Gray's Anatomy, 38th Ed., 1995, Chs.10,15.

9 a) F   also part of frontal bone and maxillae.
   b) T
   c) T
   d) T
   e) T

Gray's Anatomy, 38th Ed., 1995, Ch.11.

10 a) T
   b) F   allows easy analysis of data and trends over time.
   c) T   operating level maintained; other processes adjusted to match it.
   d) F   only the upper control limit is necessary.
   e) T

Radiographics, 1997, 17, 177-187.

Paper Four   Answers

11   a)   T
      b)   T   due to risk of aspiration.
      c)   F   colon rapidly fills with air.
      d)   F   higher incidence of missed lead points after four years of age.
      e)   T

A Guide to Radiological Procedures, Chapman & Nakielny, 3rd Ed., 1993, Ch.3.

12   a)   F   divides left lobe into medial and lateral segments.
      b)   T
      c)   F   intraperitoneal.
      d)   T
      e)   F   posterior.

Dynamic Radiology of the Abdomen, Meyers, 4th Ed., 1993, Ch.1.

13   a)   F   separated by obturator externus tendon.
      b)   T
      c)   T
      d)   F   obturator externus; internus behind.
      e)   T

Gray's Anatomy, 38th Ed., 1995, Chs.6,7.

14   a)   F
      b)   T
      c)   F
      d)   F   first generation only.
      e)   F   xenon only in later scanners.

Christensen's Physics of Diagnostic Radiology, Curry et al, 4th Ed., 1990, Ch.19.

15   a)   T
      b)   T
      c)   F   cranial angulation.
      d)   F   nearer the tube.
      e)   T

Clark's Positioning in Radiography, Swallow et al, 11th Ed., 1986, Ch.5.
Making the best use of a Department of Clinical Radiology; Royal College of Radiologists London, 2nd Ed., 1993.

Paper Four   Answers

16 a) T
  b) T
  c) T
  d) F   category A only.
  e) T

Community Radiation Protection Legislation, Commission of the European Communities, 1992.

17 a) F   contraindicated.
  b) T
  c) T
  d) F
  e) T

An Atlas of Radiological Anatomy, Weir & Abrahams, 2nd Ed., 1986.

18 a) T
  b) T
  c) F   floor of inferior horn.
  d) F   inferior frontal aspect, concerned with speech.
  e) T

Gray's Anatomy, 38th Ed., 1995, Ch.8.

19 a) F   they cross psoas major.
  b) F   upper part covered by the ligament.
  c) T
  d) T
  e) F   two origins.

Gray's Anatomy, 38th Ed., 1995, Ch.7.

20 a) F   blue and ultraviolet.
  b) T   orthochromatic film.
  c) T
  d) T   provide high contrast.
  e) T

Radiographics, 1996, 16, 1467-1479.

Paper Four Answers

21
- a) T
- b) F — better image and lower patient dose for a given tube potential.
- c) T
- d) F
- e) F — tube current and exposure time do not affect shape (quality) of spectrum.

Radiographics, 1997, 17, 967-984.

22
- a) T
- b) T
- c) T
- d) F — 3·8 milliSieverts.
- e) F — one and five minutes, and at three to four hours.

Practical Nuclear Medicine, Sharp et al, 1989, Ch.15.
Making the best use of a Department of Clinical Radiology; Royal College of Radiologists London, 2nd Ed., 1993.

23
- a) F — posterior aspect.
- b) T
- c) T
- d) T
- e) F — inferior.

Gray's Anatomy, 38th Ed., 1995, Chs.10,14.

24
- a) T — grooves the mediastinal surface of the left lung.
- b) F — behind.
- c) F — behind.
- d) T
- e) T

Gray's Anatomy, 38th Ed., 1995, Ch.10.

25
- a) T — two posterior, one anterior.
- b) F
- c) T
- d) F
- e) T — thickness in mms equates roughly with menstrual age in weeks.

Ultrasonography in Obstetrics and Gynecology, Callen, 3rd Ed., 1994, Chs.7,10,15,20.

Paper Four Answers

26
a) T
b) T
c) F
d) T
e) F

MRI made easy, Schild, 1990.

27
a) T cause a beaded appearance.
b) T more than this increases the likelihood of oily pulmonary emboli.
c) T increases if there is obstruction.
d) F L1-L2.
e) T can follow progress.

An Atlas of Radiological Anatomy, Weir & Abrahams, 2nd Ed., 1986.

28
a) F this is the AP position.
b) T
c) F axilla.
d) F supine.
e) T body of scapula parallel to film.

Clark's Positioning in Radiography, Swallow et al, 11th Ed., 1986, Ch.2.

29
a) F posterior.
b) F
c) T due to left ventricle bulging in.
d) F right considerably larger.
e) F but has thicker walls.

Gray's Anatomy, 38th Ed., 1995, Ch.10.

30
a) F log of this ratio.
b) T
c) F
d) F inverse relationship; reciprocal of exposure is a measure of speed.
e) T

Christensen's Physics of Diagnostic Radiology, Curry et al, 4th Ed., 1990, Ch.11.

Paper Four   Answers

31 a) T
    b) T
    c) F   crosses behind.
    d) F   from the upper lobe bronchus.
    e) T

Gray's Anatomy, 38th Ed., 1995, Ch.11.
A Textbook of Radiology and Imaging, Sutton, 5th Ed., 1993, Ch.11.

32 a) T   eventually pierces the clavipectoral fascia.
    b) T   right subclavian vein receives the right lymphatic duct.
    c) F   right side; inconstant.
    d) F
    e) T

Gray's Anatomy, 38th Ed., 1995, Ch.10.

33 a) T
    b) F
    c) T
    d) F   passes in front.
    e) T

Gray's Anatomy, 38th Ed., 1995, Ch.12.

34 a) T
    b) F
    c) T   reduces low energy photons more than high energy ones.
    d) F   greatest.
    e) F   can be up to 30%.

Radiographics, 1996, 16, 903-916.

35 a) F
    b) T
    c) F   distal.
    d) T
    e) T

Gray's Anatomy, 38th Ed., 1995, Ch.6.

Paper Four Answers

36
- a) T
- b) F foramen spinosum.
- c) T 0·7 to 10·4% of modern population.
- d) F foramen lacerum is not traversed by any major structures.
- e) T hypoglossal nerve, branch of ascending pharyngeal artery, emissary vein.

Gray's Anatomy, 38th Ed., 1995, Ch.6.

37
- a) F right to left shunt.
- b) T
- c) F
- d) F low energy general purpose collimator.
- e) T

Practical Nuclear Medicine, Sharp et al, 1989, Ch.10.
Making the best use of a Department of Clinical Radiology; Royal College of Radiologists London, 2nd Ed., 1993.

38
- a) T an anticholinergic side effect.
- b) F 15 minutes.
- c) T 0·3mg for barium meal.
- d) F has no effect on this.
- e) T especially in children.

A Guide to Radiological Procedures, Chapman & Nakielny, 3rd Ed., 1993, Ch.3.

39
- a) T
- b) F
- c) F
- d) F
- e) F

Techniques in Diagnostic Imaging, Whitehouse et al, 2nd Ed., 1990, Ch.24.

40
- a) F
- b) T
- c) T
- d) F
- e) F

Christensen's Physics of Diagnostic Radiology, Curry et al, 4th Ed., 1990, Ch.20.

Paper Four   Answers

41 a) F   internal carotid and posterior cerebral.
    b) T
    c) T
    d) F
    e) T

Gray's Anatomy, 38th Ed., 1995, Ch.10.

42 a) T
    b) F   lower part of head and uncinate process from ventral bud.
    c) T
    d) F   dorsal mesogastrium.
    e) T

Gray's Anatomy, 38th Ed., 1995, Ch.3.

43 a) T
    b) F   should be less than 50 micromoles/litre.
    c) F   infusion over one hour gives maximum biliary excretion.
    d) T   better duct visualisation; fewer side effects.
    e) F

A Guide to Radiological Procedures, Chapman & Nakielny, 3rd Ed., 1993, Ch.4.

44 a) T
    b) F   this is bremsstrahlung; characteristic x-rays have specific bands of energy.
    c) F   proportional to the tube potential^2.
    d) F
    e) T

Radiographics, 1997, 17, 967-984.

45 a) F   anode side.
    b) F
    c) T
    d) T
    e) F

Christensen's Physics of Diagnostic Radiology, Curry et al, 4th Ed., 1990, Ch.2.

Paper Four   Answers

46
a) F
b) F
c) T
d) T
e) F

An Atlas of Radiological Anatomy, Weir & Abrahams, 2nd Ed., 1986.

47
a) F
b) T
c) T
d) F   cords will not abduct.
e) F

An Atlas of Radiological Anatomy, Weir & Abrahams, 2nd Ed., 1986.

48
a) T
b) F
c) T
d) T
e) F   direct ratio; not log.

Christensen's Physics of Diagnostic Radiology, Curry et al, 4th Ed., 1990, Ch.14.

49
a) T
b) T
c) F
d) F
e) F

Practical Nuclear Medicine, Sharp et al, 1989, Ch.2.

50
a) T
b) F
c) F   increases number of contracted segments.
d) T
e) F   given earlier; barium seems to inhibit its action.

Techniques in Diagnostic Imaging, Whitehouse et al, 2nd Ed., 1990, Ch.3.
Pharmaco-radiology in barium examinations with special reference to glucagon, British Journal of Radiology, 1975, 48, 691-703.

Paper Four   Answers

51
a) T
b) F
c) T
d) F   but will if large collaterals are present.
e) F   but this should be drained.

A Guide to Radiological Procedures, Chapman & Nakielny, 3rd Ed., 1993, Ch.9.

52
a) T
b) T
c) F   no longer recommended.
d) T   pregnancy is a contraindication.
e) F   10 to 20mls.

A Guide to Radiological Procedures, Chapman & Nakielny, 3rd Ed., 1993, Ch.6.

53
a) T
b) F   inversely proportional to energy^3.
c) T
d) T
e) F   majority.

Christensen's Physics of Diagnostic Radiology, Curry et al, 4th Ed., 1990, Ch.4.

54
a) T
b) F   slight caudal tilt to show maximum number of ribs.
c) F   cranial tilt, 10°.
d) F   breathing diffuses lung and rib shadows.
e) T

Clark's Positioning in Radiography, Swallow et al, 11th Ed., 1986, Ch.6.

55
a) T
b) T
c) F
d) F
e) T

A Textbook of Radiology and Imaging, Sutton, 5th Ed., 1993, Ch.4.

56
a) T
b) F duct is superficial.
c) T
d) F two heads.
e) T

Gray's Anatomy, 38th Ed., 1995, Ch.7.

57
a) T
b) F
c) T
d) F
e) T

Radiographics, 1996, 16, 1165-1181.

58
a) T but decreases signal to noise.
b) T
c) F
d) T
e) T

Radiographics, 1995, 15, 683-696.

59
a) T absorbs less low energy x-rays.
b) F designed to protect bearings from heat damage.
c) F this leaks outside the housing.
d) T known as 'blooming'.
e) T

Radiographics, 1997, 17, 1259-1268.

60
a) T
b) T
c) F inspiratory and expiratory views.
d) F wood is of air attenuation at CT.
e) F

Clark's Positioning in Radiography, Swallow et al, 11th Ed., 1986, Chs.15,18.
A Textbook of Radiology and Imaging, Sutton, 6th Ed., 1997, Chs.19,49.

Paper Five

Questions

Paper Five   Questions

1 For the petrous bones

   a) the central ray passes along the orbitomeatal line in a per-orbital view.
   b) the median sagittal plane is perpendicular to the film for a Stenver's view.
   c) both sides should be examined for comparison.
   d) a large focal spot is preferred to a small one.
   e) the ossicles are usually visible on plain radiographs.

2 Coherent scatter involves

   a) loss of energy by the photon.
   b) production of ionisation.
   c) production of significant film fogging.
   d) deflection by bound electrons.
   e) a change in wavelength of the photon.

3 Myelography

   a) is contraindicated in the presence of spinal cord tumour.
   b) is contraindicated in the presence of cerebral arteriovenous malformation.
   c) is contraindicated when there has been a previous adverse reaction to intravenous iodinated contrast medium.
   d) requires prior dehydration of the patient.
   e) is best performed with a 20 gauge needle.

4 In imaging of the lymphatic system

   a) lymphangitis is common after lymphangiography.
   b) lymph vessels are best seen 24 hours after lymphangiography.
   c) lymphoscintigraphy yields high resolution anatomical detail.
   d) gallium 67 citrate does not normally accumulate in the liver.
   e) gallium 67 has a half-life of 78 hours.

5 In lower gastrointestinal investigations in children

   a) barium is used to diagnose Hirschsprung's disease.
   b) Gastrografin is used to diagnose meconium ileus.
   c) isotonic water soluble contrast medium at a height of one foot is used to diagnose site of obstruction.
   d) Gastrografin is not a cause of dehydration.
   e) reduction of an intussusception can only be performed radiologically using barium.

6 The following are true of angiographic procedures

a) haematoma occurs in all translumbar aortograms.
b) low osmolar contrast medium is preferred for peripheral angiography.
c) cobra catheters are suitable for selective angiography.
d) renal angiography typically requires 50mls of contrast medium per kidney.
e) selective head and neck angiography uses 20mls of contrast medium per vessel.

7 In the spine

a) the posterior surface of a dorsal vertebral body is almost flat.
b) the ligamentum nuchae does not attach to the skull base.
c) the dorsal spinous processes overlap.
d) the lumbar vertebral canal is round in shape.
e) the sacral canal terminates at the sacral hiatus.

8 In radiation protection

a) gloves should have a protective equivalent of at least 0·25mm lead up to 150kV.
b) body aprons should have at least 0·25mm lead equivalent for exposures up to 100kV.
c) a category A worker is one liable to receive more than 30% of one of the annual dose limits.
d) medical records of category A workers are kept for 30 years after retirement.
e) the absorbed dose rate at the patient's skin should not exceed 0·1 Gray per minute.

9 Acceptance testing

a) is the first step in quality control.
b) ensures product performance meets specifications.
c) is not applicable to cassette screens.
d) allows a base fog of 1·0 for film.
e) requires sensitometric testing for meaningful evaluation of photographic chemicals.

10 Regarding the salivary glands

a) accessory parotid gland tissue lies on the masseter muscle.
b) the facial nerve passes through the parotid gland.
c) the parotid duct passes through accessory gland tissue when this is present.
d) the submandibular gland lies completely below the mylohyoid muscle.
e) sublingual ducts enter the floor of the mouth separately.

11 Rotating anodes

a) are made of tungsten only.
b) rotate at 300 revolutions per minute.
c) are lubricated by graphite.
d) lose heat mainly by radiation.
e) have a bevel of 45 degrees.

12 In intravenous urography

a) image quality is improved by fluid restriction.
b) oral prednisolone is a reasonable precaution in an allergic patient.
c) compression is contraindicated in renal trauma.
d) myeloma is a contraindication.
e) a gas producing drink is useful in children.

13 In the head and neck

a) the anterior triangle is bounded posteriorly by the anterior border of sternocleidomastoid.
b) the posterior triangle is bounded by trapezius.
c) the submandibular gland lies completely in the digastric triangle.
d) the occipital triangle is crossed by the accessory nerve.
e) the supraclavicular triangle usually contains both the subclavian artery and vein.

14 In a barium meal examination

a) lying the patient on the left side is most likely to show gastro-oesophageal reflux.
b) the right anterior oblique position fills the fundus with barium.
c) intravenous Buscopan hinders the detection of hiatus hernia.
d) the duodenal cap is usually best shown in the right anterior oblique position.
e) colonic obstruction is a contraindication.

15 Regarding the duodenum

a) the descending duodenum lies behind the transverse colon.
b) an accessory pancreatic duct usually enters the duodenum distal to the main pancreatic duct.
c) the horizontal part of the duodenum crosses the right ureter.
d) the fourth part of the duodenum passes behind the inferior mesenteric vein.
e) the duodenal cap is the least fixed part.

16 In atomic physics

a) atomic number is the sum of the protons and neutrons in the nucleus.
b) atomic mass is the sum of the protons and electrons.
c) isotopes have the same atomic number but different atomic mass.
d) isotopes of a substance have different numbers of neutrons.
e) all isotopes of an element are radioactive to the same degree.

17 Hyoscine n-butyl bromide (Buscopan)

a) is a ganglion blocker with central action.
b) is used as a hurrying agent in small bowel studies.
c) is used both intramuscularly and intravenously.
d) has no contraindications to use.
e) is a short acting agent.

18 In emission computed tomography

a) stable distribution of radionuclide is necessary.
b) detector responses are non-uniform.
c) an accurate centre of rotation for the tomogram is not required.
d) contrast is improved by tomographic imaging.
e) images are more susceptible to artefact than conventional scintigraphy.

19 In magnetic resonance imaging

a) spin-echo sequences need only short acquisition times.
b) TR and TE control T1 and T2 weighting.
c) short TR and long TE images give poor contrast.
d) with long TR and short TE, contrast is due to proton density.
e) relaxation factors do not affect contrast.

20 In the lower limb

a) the infrapatellar bursa lies in front of the tibial tuberosity.
b) the anterior cruciate ligament attaches to the posterior aspect of the tibia.
c) the neck of the fibula is related to the common peroneal nerve.
d) the plantar ligaments attach medially on the calcaneum.
e) the base of the fifth metatarsal has no muscle attachments.

21 Regarding parotid sialography

a) standard control films should include an occlusal film.
b) Stensen's duct opens opposite the second upper molar.
c) acute infection is a contraindication.
d) 10mls of contrast medium is injected.
e) post-emptying films are of little diagnostic value.

22 Regarding x-ray generators

a) the transformer requires direct current to operate.
b) triodes contain a grid.
c) the filament circuit uses a step-up transformer.
d) the tube current is controlled by the filament current.
e) the tube current is much larger than the filament current.

23 Percutaneous transhepatic cholangiography

a) is performed with a Chiba needle.
b) is safe when the prothrombin time is five seconds longer than the control.
c) has a complication rate independent of the number of passes made.
d) results in lymphatic filling if excessive parenchymal injection occurs.
e) has morbidity and mortality of 5%.

24 In the lungs

a) the pulmonary veins closely parallel the bronchi.
b) the left main bronchus is more horizontal than the right.
c) the left main bronchus is larger than the right.
d) bronchography can be performed via cricothyroid membrane puncture.
e) the left main bronchus is longer than the right.

25 In the lower limb

a) the femoral artery lies medial to the vein in the femoral triangle.
b) the profunda femoris arises from the lateral side of the femoral artery.
c) the anterior tibial artery lies on the interosseous membrane and becomes the dorsalis pedis.
d) the peroneal artery arises from the anterior tibial artery.
e) the posterior tibial artery passes behind the medial malleolus.

Paper Five   Questions

26   In an image intensifier

   a)   the photocathode emits electrons in proportion to the intensity of the x-ray beam.
   b)   the focusing lens causes a magnified image.
   c)   the anode is at a potential of 25 to 35kV.
   d)   the output phosphor is composed of zinc cadmium sulphide.
   e)   the aluminium layer of the output screen is for structural support only.

27   The following are true of radiographic film

   a)   the polyester base measures approximately 0·2mm thick.
   b)   the base contains a dye.
   c)   the emulsion layer is typically more than 0·5mm thick.
   d)   90% of the crystals in the emulsion are silver iodide.
   e)   processing solutions weaken the gelatin layer.

28   The following are true

   a)   the normal common bile duct is up to 6mms diameter at T-tube cholangiography.
   b)   the sigmoid sinus is closely related to the mastoid antrum.
   c)   transverse horizontal folds in the rectum are most marked when the rectum is distended.
   d)   the quantity of x-rays produced is proportional to the atomic number of the target.
   e)   an occipito-frontal projection is preferable to a fronto-occipital.

29   In the upper arm

   a)   the rotator cuff comprises the fused tendons of subscapularis, supraspinatus, infraspinatus and teres minor.
   b)   the lower border of pectoralis major forms the anterior axillary fold.
   c)   the posterior axillary fold is formed by latissimus dorsi and teres minor.
   d)   the clavipectoral fascia is pierced only by the cephalic vein.
   e)   supraspinatus is separated from deltoid by the subacromial bursa.

30   In chest radiography

   a)   the normal hilar shadow contains vessels only.
   b)   the right ventricle contributes to the left heart border on a PA view.
   c)   a companion shadow lies along the inferior border of the clavicle on a PA view.
   d)   the left oblique fissure lies more anteriorly than the right on a lateral view.
   e)   on a lateral view the trachea slants anteriorly as it passes inferiorly.

31 The following are dimeric contrast media

a) iocarmate.
b) ioxaglate.
c) iotrolan.
d) iothalamate.
e) iopamidol.

32 Regarding grids

a) they stop scattered radiation but not primary beam photons.
b) the Bucky factor is only applicable to scattered radiation.
c) typical Bucky factors are from 1 to 6.
d) grid ratio is the ratio of the height to interspace width.
e) grids cause an improvement in image contrast.

33 In radiography of the sinuses

a) grids are not required.
b) the beam is perpendicular to the film for an occipito-mental view.
c) lateral views centre 2·5cms posterior to the outer canthus of the eye.
d) submentovertical views demonstrate the sphenoid and anterior ethmoid sinuses.
e) the posterior ethmoid sinuses are well shown on an optic foramen view.

34 In the subarachnoid spaces

a) the cisterna magna is continuous with the spinal subarachnoid space.
b) the basilar artery lies in the interpeduncular cistern.
c) arachnoid granulations do not affect bone.
d) communication occurs with the fourth ventricle.
e) arachnoid villi absorb cerebrospinal fluid.

35 Within the chest

a) the main pulmonary trunk lies to the left of the ascending aorta.
b) the right pulmonary artery lies in front of the superior vena cava.
c) the anterior interventricular coronary artery arises from the right coronary artery.
d) the left superior intercostal vein crosses the left side of the aortic arch.
e) the brachiocephalic artery lies behind the left brachiocephalic vein.

36 A 30° fronto-occipital skull view (Towne's) clearly shows

a) the dorsum sella.
b) the internal auditory meati.
c) the innominate lines.
d) the frontal bone.
e) the zygomatic arches.

37 Regarding MRI signal

a) T1 is the time taken to reach 63% of the original longitudinal magnetisation.
b) T2 is the time taken for transverse magnetisation to decrease to 37% of its original value.
c) T1 is one to two times longer than T2.
d) fat has a short T1 and will be bright on T1 weighted images.
e) water has a long T2 and will be bright on T2 weighted images.

38 Regarding image quality in CT

a) modern units have spatial resolution of the order of 15 line pairs per mm.
b) spatial resolution is improved at the expense of contrast resolution.
c) low contrast visibility is determined by noise.
d) only density differences of 5% or more can be detected.
e) spatial resolution is determined by pixel size.

39 Regarding ultrasound interactions

a) the acoustic impedance of a material is the product of its density and the velocity of sound within it.
b) acoustic impedance determines beam refraction.
c) as the angle of incidence increases less sound is reflected.
d) Snell's law of refraction is independent of the incident angle.
e) absorption is determined by the frequency of sound alone.

40 The larynx

a) lies between C3 and C6 in an adult male.
b) has its inlet bounded by the epiglottis and the aryepiglottic folds.
c) thyroid cartilage ceases growth at approximately twenty years of age.
d) the vestibule lies above the false cords.
e) has all its intrinsic muscles supplied by the recurrent laryngeal nerve.

Paper Five   Questions

41   In computer and information technology

a) each bit (binary digit) can represent many values.
b) bits can only represent numbers.
c) eight bits comprise a byte.
d) a network allows two or more computers to communicate.
e) bandwidth limits the amount of information sent over a data channel.

42   In the head

a) defects occur normally in the disc of the temporomandibular joint.
b) the posterior clinoid processes provide attachment for the tentorium cerebelli.
c) the frontonasal canals open into the superior meati.
d) the lacrimal gland fossa lies in the anteromedial aspect of the orbit.
e) the maxillary sinus opens into the middle meatus.

43   The following are true of radiation protection for exposed workers

a) the same dose limits apply to workers of all ages.
b) the dose limit for the lens is 300 milliSieverts (30 rems) per annum.
c) the dose limit for the skin is 500 milliSieverts (50 rems) per annum.
d) there is no dose limit for the extremities.
e) the effective dose limit is 50 milliSieverts (5 rems) per annum.

44   With regard to arthrography

a) a joint effusion should be drained prior to the procedure.
b) meglumine salts are preferable to sodium salts.
c) delayed films are of little value.
d) resorption of air and contrast medium occurs within 24 hours.
e) joint stiffness typically persists for several weeks.

45   Concerning technetium generators

a) molybdenum99 is the parent nuclide.
b) elution is performed with 0·9% saline.
c) technetium99m is safely stored and handled in lead pots of 1mm thickness.
d) radionuclide purity is not related to the radioactivity of the source.
e) radiochemical purity is the percentage of radionuclide present in the desired chemical form.

46 The sternoclavicular joints

a) are obscured by the spine on an AP projection.
b) require oblique views for clear visualisation.
c) are best shown with patient's median sagittal plane perpendicular to the film.
d) require suspended respiration during the exposure.
e) should both be examined routinely.

47 The following are true of the ureters

a) the abdominal portions cross anterior to the gonadal veins.
b) they enter the pelvis anterior to the common iliac termination.
c) the narrowest segment is at the pelvic brim.
d) in the male, they are crossed anterosuperiorly by the vas.
e) they receive blood supply from the aorta and iliac vessels only.

48 Regarding Potter-Bucky (moving) grids

a) they move continuously during the exposure.
b) they have no effect on the appearance of grid lines on the film.
c) their use causes an increase in patient dose.
d) they are a cause of lateral decentering.
e) they do not affect the duration of exposure.

49 Regarding the testis and epididymis

a) the testis is completely surrounded by the tunica vaginalis.
b) the epididymis lies posterolaterally.
c) the appendix of the epididymis arises from the tail.
d) the testicular arteries lie anterior to the external iliac arteries.
e) lymphatic drainage is to the inguinal nodes.

50 The following are true of mediastinal structures

a) the superior mediastinum lies between the manubrium sternum and the upper four thoracic vertebrae.
b) the anterior mediastinum contains no vessels.
c) the posterior mediastinum lies anterior to the fourth to twelfth dorsal vertebrae.
d) on a PA chest x-ray, the inferior vena cava contributes to the right mediastinal contour.
e) in a child the thymus may have an enlarged appearance with a wavy outline.

51 Range-gated (pulsed) Doppler ultrasound

a) allows spatial (depth) resolution.
b) requires pulse repetition frequency to be at least twice the frequency of interest.
c) increasing pulse repetition frequency decreases aliasing.
d) as scan angle approaches 90° motion of the vessel wall confuses flow signal.
e) lower carrier (interrogation) frequencies produce lower Doppler shifts.

52 In radiography of the elbow

a) the AP beam is centred 2·5cms distal to the midpoint of the epicondyles.
b) lateral views are obtained with the shoulder and elbow at the same level.
c) the radial head is more clearly seen in supination on a lateral view.
d) the proximal radio-ulnar joint is seen in the oblique position.
e) a modified axial view in partial flexion will show the ulnar groove.

53 In the cerebral hemispheres

a) the interventricular foramen lies at the level of the mid-body of the lateral ventricles.
b) the head of the caudate nucleus forms the floor of the anterior horn of the lateral ventricle.
c) the posterior horns of the lateral ventricles are almost always symmetrical.
d) the caudate nucleus lies medial to the posterior limb of the internal capsule.
e) the lentiform nucleus comprises the putamen and globus pallidus.

54 Limiting resolution

a) is the number of line pairs per mm identifiable in an image of a bar test object.
b) is affected by subject contrast.
c) is not affected by film contrast.
d) is not affected by blur.
e) is affected by noise.

55 In MRI of the spine

a) the nucleus pulposus has a high signal on T2 weighted images.
b) the annulus fibrosis has a low signal on T2 weighted images.
c) cerebrospinal fluid has a low signal on T1 weighted images.
d) differentiation of cortex and medulla of bone is not possible.
e) the nerve roots are not clearly visualised.

Paper Five   Questions

56 The pituitary gland

    a)   is not covered by meninges.
    b)   is connected to the thalamus by the infundibulum.
    c)   is separated from the floor of the pituitary fossa by a venous sinus.
    d)   is supplied by a single inferior and several superior hypophyseal arteries.
    e)   is approximately 2cms in transverse diameter.

57 In ultrasound during pregnancy

    a)   foetal cardiac pulsation should be visible when the crown-rump length is 5mms.
    b)   the foetal head can be distinguished from the torso when the crown-rump length is approximately 8mms.
    c)   the crown-rump length is the most accurate assessor of foetal age in the first trimester.
    d)   the corpus luteum cyst regresses at the end of the first trimester.
    e)   an uncomplicated corpus luteum cyst is almost always thin walled.

58 Regarding image quality

    a)   film graininess has a significant effect on radiographic mottle.
    b)   quantum mottle is caused by the statistical fluctuation in the number of photons absorbed per unit area.
    c)   quantum mottle is not seen when intensifying screens are used.
    d)   fast screens increase unsharpness.
    e)   low contrast images are limited by noise.

59 In macro-radiography

    a)   the focus to film distance is increased.
    b)   the object to film distance is increased.
    c)   photographic unsharpness is increased.
    d)   a large focal spot is needed to increase magnification and maintain quality.
    e)   scatter is reduced.

60 With regard to the fallopian tubes and broad ligament

    a)   the fallopian tubes lie in the central portion of the broad ligaments.
    b)   in the nulliparous state, the fallopian tubes cross anterior to the ovary.
    c)   the fallopian tubes are the commonest site for an ectopic pregnancy.
    d)   the isthmus is the widest segment of the fallopian tube.
    e)   injection of contrast medium into the uterus will spill into the peritoneal cavity.

Paper Five

Answers

Paper Five   Answers

1.
   a) T
   b) F   approximately 45°.
   c) T
   d) F   0·6mm or less.
   e) F

Clark's Positioning in Radiography, Swallow et al, 11th Ed., 1986, Ch.8.

2.
   a) F
   b) F
   c) F   insignificant amounts at diagnostic energies.
   d) T
   e) F   change of direction only.

Christensen's Physics of Diagnostic Radiology, Curry et al, 4th Ed., 1990, Ch.4.

3.
   a) F
   b) T
   c) F
   d) F   should be avoided.
   e) F   22 gauge.

A Guide to Radiological Procedures, Chapman & Nakielny, 3rd Ed., 1993, Ch.12.

4.
   a) F
   b) F   lymph nodes; vessels have emptied.
   c) F
   d) F
   e) T

A Guide to Radiological Procedures, Chapman & Nakielny, 3rd Ed., 1993, Ch.10.

5.
   a) T
   b) T
   c) T
   d) F
   e) F   also air.

Techniques in Diagnostic Imaging, Whitehouse et al, 2nd Ed., 1990, Ch.24.

Paper Five   Answers

6   a)   T
    b)   T
    c)   T
    d)   F   less than 10mls per kidney.
    e)   F   less than 10mls.

A Guide to Radiological Procedures, Chapman & Nakielny, 3rd Ed., 1993, Ch.8.

7   a)   T   or minimally concave.
    b)   F
    c)   T
    d)   F   triangular.
    e)   T

Gray's Anatomy, 38th Ed., 1995, Ch.6.

8   a)   T
    b)   T   0 to 100 kV, 0·25mm; 100 to 150 kV, 0·35mm.
    c)   T
    d)   T
    e)   T

Community Radiation Protection Legislation, Commission of the European Communities, 1992.

9   a)   T
    b)   T
    c)   F   should assess speed uniformity.
    d)   F   0·03.
    e)   T

Radiographics, 1997, 17, 177-187.

10   a)   T
     b)   T
     c)   F   lies inferior to accessory tissue.
     d)   F   deep part lies above.
     e)   T

Gray's Anatomy, 38th Ed., 1995, Ch.12.

Paper Five   Answers

11 a) **F** tungsten embedded in copper with a molybdenum stem.
    b) **F** 3000 revolutions per minute.
    c) **F** silver.
    d) **T**
    e) **F** 6 to 20 degrees.

Christensen's Physics of Diagnostic Radiology, Curry et al, 4th Ed., 1990, Ch.2.

12 a) **F**
    b) **T** 32mgs methyl prednisolone orally 12 and 2 hours before injection.
    c) **T**
    d) **F** myeloma is a contraindication to dehydration, not urography.
    e) **T** allows a window through the stomach.

A Guide to Radiological Procedures, Chapman & Nakielny, 3rd Ed., 1993, Ch.5.

13 a) **T**
    b) **T**
    c) **F** lies partly above mylohyoid.
    d) **T**
    e) **F** artery only, vein occasionally.

Gray's Anatomy, 38th Ed., 1995, Ch.10.

14 a) **F**
    b) **T**
    c) **F**
    d) **T**
    e) **T** especially if complete.

A Guide to Radiological Procedures, Chapman & Nakielny, 3rd Ed., 1993, Ch.3.

15 a) **T**
    b) **F** usually proximal.
    c) **T**
    d) **F** in front.
    e) **T** rest relatively fixed.

Gray's Anatomy, 38th Ed., 1995, Ch.12.

Paper Five   Answers

16 a) F   protons only.
    b) F   sum of protons and neutrons.
    c) T
    d) T
    e) F

Radiographics, 1997, 17, 967-984.

17 a) F   no central action.
    b) F   no effect on motility.
    c) T
    d) F
    e) T

*Techniques in Diagnostic Imaging, Whitehouse et al, 2nd Ed., 1990, Ch.3.
Pharmaco-radiology in barium examinations with special reference to glucagon,
British Journal of Radiology, 1975, 48, 691-703.*

18 a) T
    b) F   uniform detector response is necessary.
    c) F
    d) T
    e) T

Radiographics, 1995, 15, 975-991.

19 a) F   need long times (1 to 10 minutes).
    b) T
    c) T   should be avoided; also have low signal to noise ratio.
    d) T
    e) F

Radiographics, 1994, 14, 1389-1404.

20 a) T
    b) F   anterior.
    c) T   crosses lateral neck below the head of the fibula.
    d) F   on lateral aspect of the plantar surface.
    e) F

Gray's Anatomy, 38th Ed., 1995, Ch.6.

Paper Five   Answers

21 a) F
    b) T
    c) T
    d) F   less than 2mls usually.
    e) F

A Textbook of Radiology and Imaging, Sutton, 6th Ed., 1997, Ch.28.
A Guide to Radiological Procedures, Chapman & Nakielny, 3rd Ed., 1993, Ch.14.

22 a) F   alternating, in order to produce a changing magnetic field.
    b) T
    c) F   step-down.
    d) T
    e) F   much smaller (tube 1 to 1000mA; filament 1 to 10Amps).

Radiographics, 1997, 17, 1533-1557.

23 a) T
    b) F   two seconds greater.
    c) T
    d) T
    e) F   morbidity 5%, mortality less than 0·1%.

A Guide to Radiological Procedures, Chapman & Nakielny, 3rd Ed., 1993, Ch.4.

24 a) F   arteries parallel bronchi.
    b) T
    c) F
    d) T
    e) T

An Atlas of Radiological Anatomy, Weir & Abrahams, 2nd Ed., 1986.

25 a) F
    b) T   then courses behind and medially.
    c) T
    d) F   posterior tibial.
    e) T

Gray's Anatomy, 38th Ed., 1995, Ch.10.

Paper Five   Answers

26 a) T
    b) F   minified; also inverted.
    c) T
    d) T
    e) F   prevents retrograde travel of light.

Christensen's Physics of Diagnostic Radiology, Curry et al, 4th Ed., 1990, Ch.12.

27 a) T
    b) T
    c) F   thinner.
    d) F   90% bromide.
    e) F   gelatin retains strength and permanence.

Christensen's Physics of Diagnostic Radiology, Curry et al, 4th Ed., 1990, Ch.10.

28 a) F   12mms.
    b) T   separated by a thin plate of bone.
    c) T
    d) T
    e) T   reduces eye dose.

Gray's Anatomy, 38th Ed., 1995, Chs.10,12.
Radiographics, 1997, 17, 967-984.
Clark's Positioning in Radiography, Swallow et al, 11th Ed., 1986, Ch.8.
An Atlas of Radiological Anatomy, Weir & Abrahams, 1986, 2nd Ed..

29 a) T
    b) T
    c) F   teres major.
    d) F   also thoraco-acromial vessels and lateral pectoral nerve.
    e) T

Gray's Anatomy, 38th Ed., 1995, Ch.7.

30 a) T
    b) F
    c) F   superior.
    d) F
    e) F   posteriorly.

An Atlas of Radiological Anatomy, Weir & Abrahams, 2nd Ed., 1986.

Paper Five   Answers

31
a) T
b) T
c) T
d) F
e) F

Techniques in Diagnostic Imaging, Whitehouse et al, 2nd Ed., 1990, Ch.30.

32
a) F
b) F represents overall reduction in x-ray intensity produced by grid.
c) T
d) T
e) T

Radiographics, 1996, 16, 903-916.

33
a) F
b) T
c) T
d) F sphenoids and posterior ethmoids.
e) T

Clark's Positioning in Radiography, Swallow et al, 11th Ed., 1986, Ch.9.

34
a) T
b) F pontine.
c) F cause resorption and produce small pits.
d) T via median and lateral apertures.
e) T

Gray's Anatomy, 38th Ed., 1995, Ch.8.

35
a) T
b) F
c) F
d) T
e) T

Gray's Anatomy, 38th Ed., 1995, Ch.10.

Paper Five   Answers

36
a) T   projected into foramen magnum if positioning is correct.
b) T
c) F
d) F
e) T

An Atlas of Radiological Anatomy, Weir & Abrahams, 2nd Ed., 1986.

37
a) T
b) T
c) F   2·5 to 10 times longer.
d) T
e) T

MRI made easy, Schild, 1990.

38
a) F   15 line pairs/cm.
b) T
c) T
d) F   0·5%.
e) T   also scanner design, display unit.

Christensen's Physics of Diagnostic Radiology, Curry et al, 4th Ed., 1990, Ch.19.

39
a) T
b) F   beam reflection.
c) T
d) F
e) F   also viscosity, relaxation time of material.

Christensen's Physics of Diagnostic Radiology, Curry et al, 4th Ed., 1990, Ch.20.

40
a) T
b) T
c) F   40 years in men.
d) T
e) F   cricothyroid supplied by the external laryngeal nerve.

Gray's Anatomy, 38th Ed., 1995, Ch.11.

Paper Five   Answers

41
- a) F — only two values, e.g. on or off; often represented by 1 and 0.
- b) F — also letters, image data etc..
- c) T
- d) T
- e) T

Radiographics, 1997, 17, 985-992.

42
- a) T
- b) T
- c) F — middle meati.
- d) F — anterolateral.
- e) T

Gray's Anatomy, 38th Ed., 1995, Ch.6.

43
- a) F — under 18s can only receive 30% of the annual limit.
- b) T
- c) T
- d) F — limit of 500 milliSieverts per annum.
- e) T

Community Radiation Protection Legislation, Commission of the European Communities, 1992.

44
- a) T
- b) T
- c) F
- d) F — contrast medium absorbed in hours; air in 1-2 days.
- e) F

A Guide to Radiological Procedures, Chapman & Nakielny, 3rd Ed., 1993, Ch.11.

45
- a) T
- b) T
- c) F — 3mms minimum.
- d) F
- e) T

Practical Nuclear Medicine, Sharp et al, 1989, Ch.6.

Paper Five   Answers

46
a) T
b) T
c) F   45°.
d) F   breathing blurs out lung detail.
e) T   for comparison.

Clark's Positioning in Radiography, Swallow et al, 11th Ed., 1986, Ch.2.

47
a) F   lie posterior.
b) T
c) F   bladder wall.
d) T
e) F   supply via aorta, renal, iliac, vesical, gonadal and uterine arteries.

Gray's Anatomy, 38th Ed., 1995, Ch.13.

48
a) T
b) F
c) T
d) T
e) F   they limit the minimum exposure time.

Christensen's Physics of Diagnostic Radiology, Curry et al, 4th Ed., 1990, Ch.8.

49
a) F   not completely posteriorly.
b) T
c) T
d) T
e) F

Gray's Anatomy, 38th Ed., 1995, Chs.10,14.

50
a) T
b) F   branches of internal thoracic artery.
c) T
d) T
e) T   wave sign of Mulvey.

Gray's Anatomy, 38th Ed., 1995, Ch.11.
A Textbook of Radiology and Imaging, Sutton, 5th Ed., 1993, Ch.11.

Paper Five   Answers

51 a) T
    b) T   to prevent aliasing.
    c) T
    d) T   should not go above 70°.
    e) T   and less aliasing.

Radiographics, 1994, 14, 139-150.

52 a) T
    b) T
    c) F   pronation.
    d) T
    e) F   full flexion.

Clark's Positioning in Radiography, Swallow et al, 11th Ed., 1986, Ch.1.

53 a) F   junction of frontal horns and central part.
    b) T
    c) F   often asymmetrical; may be absent.
    d) F   anterior limb.
    e) T

Gray's Anatomy, 38th Ed., 1995, Ch.8.

54 a) T
    b) T
    c) F
    d) F
    e) T

Radiographics, 1996, 16, 1165-1181.

55 a) T
    b) T
    c) T
    d) F
    e) F

A Textbook of Radiology and Imaging, Sutton, 6th Ed., 1997, Ch.55.

Paper Five   Answers

56
a) F   meninges blend with capsule.
b) F   infundibulum connects to tuber cinereum of hypothalamus.
c) T
d) T
e) F

Gray's Anatomy, 38th Ed., 1995, Ch.15.
A Textbook of Radiology and Imaging, Sutton, 5th Ed., 1993, Ch.53.

57
a) T   in all live foetuses.
b) F   12mms approximately.
c) T
d) T
e) F   often thick walled.

Ultrasonography in Obstetrics and Gynecology, Callen, 3rd Ed., 1994, Ch.6.

58
a) F
b) T
c) F
d) T
e) T

Christensen's Physics of Diagnostic Radiology, Curry et al, 4th Ed., 1990, Ch.14.

59
a) T   focus-object distance constant; film further from focus.
b) T
c) F   but movement and geometric unsharpness are.
d) F   small focal spot gives less penumbra.
e) T   due to air gap.

Clark's Positioning in Radiography, Swallow et al, 11th Ed., 1986, Ch.20.

60
a) F   upper border.
b) T
c) T
d) F
e) T

Gray's Anatomy, 38th Ed., 1995, Ch.14.

Paper Five Answers

51
a) T
b) T to prevent aliasing.
c) T
d) T should not go above 70°.
e) T and less aliasing.

Radiographics, 1994, 14, 139-150.

52
a) T
b) T
c) F pronation.
d) T
e) F full flexion.

Clark's Positioning in Radiography, Swallow et al, 11th Ed., 1986, Ch.1.

53
a) F junction of frontal horns and central part.
b) T
c) F often asymmetrical; may be absent.
d) F anterior limb.
e) T

Gray's Anatomy, 38th Ed., 1995, Ch.8.

54
a) T
b) T
c) F
d) F
e) T

Radiographics, 1996, 16, 1165-1181.

55
a) T
b) T
c) T
d) F
e) F

A Textbook of Radiology and Imaging, Sutton, 6th Ed., 1997, Ch.55.

Paper Five   Answers

56
a) F — meninges blend with capsule.
b) F — infundibulum connects to tuber cinereum of hypothalamus.
c) T
d) T
e) F

Gray's Anatomy, 38th Ed., 1995, Ch.15.
A Textbook of Radiology and Imaging, Sutton, 5th Ed., 1993, Ch.53.

57
a) T — in all live foetuses.
b) F — 12mms approximately.
c) T
d) T
e) F — often thick walled.

Ultrasonography in Obstetrics and Gynecology, Callen, 3rd Ed., 1994, Ch.6.

58
a) F
b) T
c) F
d) T
e) T

Christensen's Physics of Diagnostic Radiology, Curry et al, 4th Ed., 1990, Ch.14.

59
a) T — focus-object distance constant; film further from focus.
b) T
c) F — but movement and geometric unsharpness are.
d) F — small focal spot gives less penumbra.
e) T — due to air gap.

Clark's Positioning in Radiography, Swallow et al, 11th Ed., 1986, Ch.20.

60
a) F — upper border.
b) T
c) T
d) F
e) T

Gray's Anatomy, 38th Ed., 1995, Ch.14.